NEVER FINISHED

CLEAN EDITION

NEVER FINISHED

UNSHACKLE YOUR MIND AND WIN THE WAR WITHIN

DAVID GOGGINS

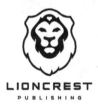

LIONCREST

PUBLISHING

NEVER FINISHED
Unshackle Your Mind and Win the War Within - Clean Edition

FIRST EDITION

ISBN 978-1-5445-3682-8 Paperback
      978-1-5445-3681-1 Ebook

TO MY NORTH STAR THAT HAS ALWAYS
SHINED, EVEN ON THE DARKEST OF NIGHTS.

CONTENTS

WARNING ORDER

TIME ZONE: 24/7

TASK ORGANIZATION: SOLO MISSION

1. SITUATION: Your horizons have been limited by societal and self-imposed barriers.

2. MISSION: Fight through resistance. Seek unknown territory. Redefine what's possible.

3. EXECUTION:

    a. Read this book cover to cover. Absorb the philosophy within. Test all theories to the best of your ability. Repeat. Repetition will sharpen new skills and stimulate growth.

    b. This will not be easy. To succeed, you will be required to face hard truths and challenge yourself like never before. This mission is about embracing and learning the lessons from each and every Evolution so you can discover who you really are and can become.

    c. Self-mastery is an unending process. Your job is NEVER FINISHED!

4. CLASSIFIED: The real work is unseen. Your performance matters most when nobody is watching.

BY COMMAND OF: DAVID GOGGINS

SIGNED:

RANK AND SERVICE: CHIEF, U.S. NAVY SEALS, RETIRED

INTRODUCTION

T his is not a self-help book. Nobody needs another sermon about the ten steps or seven stages or sixteen hours a week that will deliver them from their stalled or jacked-up life. Hit the local bookstore or surf Amazon and you will slip into a bottomless pit of self-help hype. Must feel good to consume because it sure does sell.

Too bad most of it won't work. Not for real. Not forever. You might see progress here and there, but if you are broken like I used to be or stuck wandering an endless plateau while your true potential wastes away, books alone can't and won't fix you.

Self-help is a fancy term for self-improvement, and while we should always strive to be better, improvement is often not enough. There are times in life when we become so disconnected from ourselves that we must drill down and rewire those cut connections in our hearts, minds, and souls. Because that is the only way to rediscover and reignite *belief*—that flicker in the darkness with the power to spark your evolution.

Belief is a gritty, potent, primordial force. In the 1950s, a scientist named Dr. Curt Richter proved this when he gathered dozens of rats and dropped them into thirty-inch-deep glass cylinders filled with water. The first rat paddled on the surface for a short time, then swam to the bottom, where it looked for an escape hatch. It died within two minutes. Several others followed that same pattern. Some lasted as long as fifteen minutes, but they all gave up. Richter was surprised because rats are good swimmers, yet in his lab, they drowned without much of a fight. So, he tweaked the test.

After he placed the next batch in their jars, Richter watched them, and right before it looked like they were about to give up, he and his techs scooped up the rats, toweled them off, and held them long enough for their heart and respiratory rates to normalize. Long enough for them to register, on a physiological scale, that they had been saved. They did this a few times before Richter placed a group of them back into those evil cylinders again to see how long they would last on their own. This time, the rats didn't give up. They swam their hearts out...for an average of sixty hours without any food or rest. One swam for eighty-one hours.

In his report, Richter suggested that the first round of subjects gave up because they were hopeless and that the second batch persisted for so long because they knew it was possible someone would come along and save them. The popular analysis these days is that Richter's interventions flipped a switch in the rat brain, which illuminated the power of hope for us all to see.

I love this experiment, but hope isn't what got into those

rats. How long does hope really last? It may have triggered something initially, but no creature is going to swim for their life for sixty hours straight, without food, powered by hope alone. They needed something a lot stronger to keep them breathing, kicking, and fighting.

When mountaineers tackle the tallest peaks and steepest faces, they are usually tethered to a rope fixed to anchors in the ice or rock so when they slip, they don't slide off the mountain and tumble to their deaths. They may fall ten or twelve feet, then get up, dust themselves off, and try again. Life is the mountain we are all climbing, but hope is not an anchor point. It's too soft, fluffy, and fleeting. There's no substance behind hope. It's not a muscle you can develop, and it's not rooted down deep. It's an emotion that comes and goes.

Richter touched something in his rats that was nearly unbreakable. He may not have noticed them adapting to their life-or-death trial, but they had to have figured out a more efficient technique to preserve energy. With each passing minute, they became more and more resilient until they started to believe that they would survive. Their confidence didn't fade as the hours piled up; it actually grew. They weren't hoping to be saved. They refused to die! The way I see it, belief is what turned ordinary lab rats into marine mammals.

There are two levels to belief. There's the surface level, which our coaches, teachers, therapists, and parents love to preach. "Believe in yourself," they all say, as if the thought alone can keep us afloat when the odds are against us in the battle of our lives. But once exhaustion sets in, doubt and insecurity tend to penetrate and dissipate that flimsy brand of belief.

Then there's the belief born in resilience. It comes from working your way through layers of pain, fatigue, and reason, and ignoring the ever-present temptation to quit until you strike a source of fuel you didn't even know existed. One that eliminates all doubt, makes you certain of your strength and the fact that eventually, you will prevail, so long as you keep moving forward. That is the level of belief that can defy the expectations of scientists and change everything. It's not an emotion to be shared or an intellectual concept, and nobody else can give it to you. It must bubble up from within.

When you are lost at sea and no one is coming to save you, there are only two options. You will either swim hard and figure out how to last as long as it takes, or you are bound to drown. I was born with holes in my heart and sickle cell trait, and into a childhood torched by toxic stress and learning disabilities. I had minimal potential, and by the time I turned twenty-four, I knew I was in danger of wasting my life.

Many people get it twisted and think my accomplishments directly correlate to my potential. My accomplishments do not equate to my potential. The little bit I had was buried so deep, most people would never have found it. Not only did I find it, I learned to maximize it.

I knew that there could be so much more to my story than the wreckage I saw around me, and that it was time to decide if I had it in me to go as hard as I could for as long as it took to become a more self-empowered human being. I fought through doubt and insecurity. I wanted to quit every single day, but eventually, belief kicked in. I believed I could evolve, and that same belief has given me the strength and focus to persevere whenever I've been challenged for over two decades. More often than not, I've challenged myself to see how far I can push it and how many more chapters I can add to my story. I'm still seeking new territory, still curious just how high I might rise from the bottom of the barrel.

A lot of folks feel like they are missing something in their lives—something money can't buy—and that makes them miserable. They attempt to fill the void with material things they can see, feel, and touch. But that empty feeling won't go away. It fades some until all gets quiet again. Then that familiar gnawing in their gut returns, reminding them that the life they are living is not the fullest expression of who they are or might become.

Unfortunately, most people are not desperate enough to do anything about it. When you're hogtied in conflicting emotions and other people's opinions, it's impossible to tap into belief and easy to drift away from that urge to evolve. You could be itchy to experience something different, to be somewhere different, or to become someone different, but when the slightest resistance arises to challenge your resolve, you moonwalk right back into the unsatisfied person you were before. Still itchy, still jonesing to be someone new, yet still trapped in your unfulfilling status quo. And you are nowhere near alone.

Social media has compounded and spread this virus of dissatisfaction, which is why the world is now populated by damaged people consuming airy gratification, hunting an immediate dopamine fix with no substance at all behind it. Instead of staying focused on growth, millions of minds have been infected with lack, leaving them feeling even lesser than. Their internal dialogue becomes that much more toxic, as this population of weak, entitled victims of life itself multiplies.

It's funny, we question so many things about the way our lives are going. We wonder what it would be like if we looked different, had more of a head start, or were given a boost at one time or another. Very few people question their own warped minds. Instead, they collect slights, dramas, and problems, hoarding them until they are bloated with stale regret and envy, which form the roadblocks stopping them from becoming their truest, most capable selves.

All over the world, hundreds of millions of people choose to live that way. But there is another way of thinking and another way of being. It helped me regain control of my life. It allowed me to eviscerate all obstacles in my path until my growth factor became near limitless. I'm still haunted, but I've traded in my demons for evil angels, and now, it's a good haunting. I'm haunted by my future goals, not my past failures. I'm haunted by what I may still become. I'm haunted by my own continued thirst for evolution.

The work is often as miserable and thankless as it ever was, and although there are techniques and skills I've developed that can help along the way, there is no certain number of principles, hours, or steps in this process. It's about constant effort, learning, and adaptation, which demands unwavering discipline and belief. The kind that looks a lot like desperation. See, I am the lab rat who refused to die! And I'm here to show you how to get to the other side of hell.

Most theories on performance and possibility are hatched in the controlled environment of a sterile laboratory and spread in university lecture halls. But I am not a theorist. I am a practitioner. Similar to how the late, great Stephen Hawking explored the dark matter of the universe, I am intensely passionate about exploring the dark matter of the mind—all of our untapped energy, capacity, and power. My philosophy has been tested and proven in my own Mental Lab through all the many trials and tribulations that shaped my life in the real world.

After each chapter, you will find an Evolution. In the military, evolutions are drills, exercises, or practices meant to sharpen your skills. In this book, they are hard truths we should all face, and philosophies and strategies you can use to overcome whatever is in your way—and excel in life.

Like I said, this is definitely not a self-help book. This is boot camp for your brain. It's a what-are-you-doing-with-your-life book. It's the wake-up call you don't want and probably didn't even know you needed.

Rise up!

Time to get to work!

CHAPTER ONE

MAXIMIZE MINIMAL POTENTIAL

I sat among thousands of combat veterans in a packed Kansas City Convention Center for the 2018 Veterans of Foreign Wars (VFW) National Convention. I wasn't just an active member; I was their guest. I'd been flown in to receive the VFW's prestigious Americanism Award—an annual honor for those who demonstrate a commitment to service, patriotism, the betterment of American society, and helping fellow veterans. The most famous past recipient was one of my heroes. Senator John McCain survived five and a half years as a POW during the Vietnam War. I've always admired the courage he exemplified back then, and throughout his very public life, he continued to set the standard for how I believe men should handle hard times. Now my name was going to be alongside his.

I was about to receive the greatest honor of my life so far. I should have been proud as hell. Instead, I was mystified. For over an hour, I sat in the audience between my mother, Jackie, and my uncle, John Gardner. That's a lot of time to contemplate the meaning of the moment, and all I could come up with were the reasons that I shouldn't be there. That nobody should know the name David Goggins, much less put me in the same sentence as Senator McCain. Not because I didn't earn my spot, but because the circumstances that life served me should never have led me here.

Sure, I'm a winner now, but I was born a loser. There are a lot of born losers out there. Every day, babies are born into poverty and broken families, like I was. Some lose their parents in accidents. Others are abused and neglected. Many of us are born with disabilities, some physical, others mental or emotional.

It's as if every human being is issued their own personal piñata just for making it out of the womb alive. No one gets a sneak preview of what's in their piñata, but whatever it is will set them up one way or another. Some of us smack it open and sweet things rain down. Those are the ones who have it relatively easy—at least at first. Some are empty as a dry well. Others are worse than empty. They're packed with nightmares, and the haunting begins as soon as the baby takes its first breath. That was me. I was born into a terror dome.

As the speakers took their turns on the mic, I was deep in my own dark cave, reliving the countless bloody beatings my father dealt to my mother, my brother, and me. I watched us escape to Brazil, Indiana, only to settle just ten miles from an active chapter of the Ku Klux Klan. And guess where they sent their kids to school? I recalled the steady flow of racist threats from some of my classmates and how I cheated my way through school and learned nothing.

I thought of my mother's fiancé, Wilmoth, a would-be father figure who was murdered before he could become my stepdad. I recalled my repeated attempts at the Armed Services Vocational Aptitude Battery (ASVAB), a standardized test required for all military recruits, to fulfill my dream of becoming a Pararescueman. After I finally passed that dreaded test and enlisted, I quit Pararescue training when the water evolutions became too hard. That brilliant decision ultimately led to me becoming a three-hundred-pound graveyard-shift exterminator at Ecolab, raking in $1,000 a month at twenty-four years old.

I was a shell of a man at that point, with no self-esteem or self-respect. I was still haunted by the same old demons that had tailed me from birth, and the harsh reality was that I lacked everything I needed to become the man I wanted to be.

Mind you, I wasn't thinking about all of that to punish myself. I was sifting through the files, searching for the catalyst, the moment that restarted the fire and ignited something primal inside me. I needed to remember exactly how and when I flipped the script and managed to build a life of honor and service, but I kept coming up empty. I was so deep in my brain cave I didn't even hear them call my name. I wouldn't have reacted at all if my mom hadn't nudged my arm. Even now, I don't remember walking up the stage steps with her because I was still floating between my past and my disorienting present.

I heard them read my résumé, detailing the money I'd raised for veteran causes and the objectives I'd met over the course of my career. Before I knew it, they put a medal around my neck and the audience was on their feet applauding. That was the surest sign yet that this born loser had been reborn somewhere along the way. That there had been a moment that sparked my metamorphosis.

When it was my turn at the microphone, I gazed out at all the unfamiliar faces. Members of a brotherhood and sisterhood that I will always be a part of. The fact that this recognition came from them was the deepest honor, but I didn't know how to thank them. I was a sought-after public speaker by then, comfortable in front of crowds large and small. Factor in my work as a recruiter for the military, and I'd been a professional public speaker for over a decade. I rarely got butterflies, but that summer day in Kansas City, I was nervous as hell and my mind was still clouded. I tried to shake it off and started by thanking my grandfather, Sergeant Jack.

"He would be the proudest man in the world to see me up here right now," I said. Choked up, I paused, took a deep breath to compose myself, and started again. "I'd like to thank my mom, who..." I turned to my mother, and when our eyes met, the moment that permanently changed my life finally hit me, and the power of that realization was overwhelming. "I'd like to thank my mom, who..."

My voice cracked again. I couldn't hold back the flood any longer. I closed my eyes and sobbed. Like a dream that only lasts seconds yet feels like hours, time stretched out and scenes from the ultimate turning point in my life—the last time I ever saw my father—colonized my mind. If I hadn't taken that trip, you'd never have heard of me.

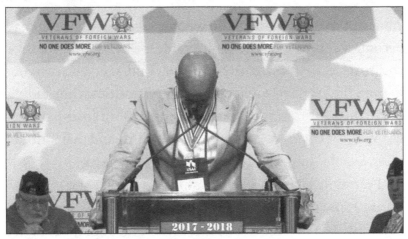

It finally hit me and I was overwhelmed by the work it took to get here.

❧ ❧ ❧

I was twenty-four years old when I realized I was broken inside. Something had gone numb in my soul, and that numbness, that lack of deep feeling, dictated what my life had become. It's why I quit going after my goals, my biggest dreams, whenever things got hard. Quitting was just another detour. It never bothered me much because when you're numb, you can't process what's happening to you or within you. I didn't know the power of the mind yet, and because of that I had ballooned into a fat boy and taken a job as a cockroach sniper in restaurants.

I had my excuses, of course. My numbness was a survival mechanism. It had been beaten into me by my father. By the time I'd turned seven, I'd developed a POW mindset. Going numb was how I took my beatings and maintained some level of self-respect. Even after my mother and I escaped, I continued to be stalked by tragedy and failure, and numbness was how I coped with the fact that losing was all I ever knew.

When you're born a loser, your goal is to survive, not thrive.

You learn to lie, to cheat, to do what it takes to fit in. You may become a survivor, but it's a miserable existence. Just like the cockroaches I was assigned to kill, you find yourself scurrying in from the shadows to claim the bare necessities while hiding your true self from the light at all costs. Born losers are the ultimate cockroaches. We do what we have to, and that attitude often enables some pretty severe character defects.

I certainly had some. I was a quitter, a liar, fat and lazy, and I was deeply depressed. I could feel myself unraveling a little at a time. Fed up and frustrated, bitter and angry, I couldn't take much more of my sorry excuse for a life. If I didn't change, and change soon, I knew I would die a loser, or worse. I might end up like my father, the hustler who was one quick twitch away from violence. I was consumed by misery and groping for some mental foothold to keep me from giving up for good. The only thing I could come up with was to go back to that house on Paradise Road that still haunted me. I had to get to Buffalo, New York, and look my father in the eye. Because when you're living in hell, the only way to find your way out is to confront the Devil himself.

I was hoping to find some answers that would help me change my life. That was what I told myself, anyway, as I crossed into Ohio from Indiana and veered northeast. I hadn't seen my old man in twelve years. It had been my decision to stop seeing him. At that time, the court system allowed children to make those decisions once they turned twelve. I made that choice mostly out of respect for and loyalty to my mom. He'd stopped beating us after we left Buffalo, but the one thing that never went numb was how I felt about what my mother endured at his hands. Still, over the years, I had questioned that decision and began to wonder if my memories, if the stories I told myself, were true.

On the long drive, I didn't listen to music. All I heard were the competing voices in my head. The first voice accepted me as I was.

It's not your fault, David. None of this is your fault. You're doing the best you can with what you've been given.

That was the voice I'd been listening to my entire life. *It's not my fault* was my favorite refrain. It explained and justified my lot in life and the dead-end path in front of me, and it played 24/7. However, for the first time, another voice chimed in. Or maybe it was the first time I stopped listening only to what I wanted to hear.

Roger that. It ain't your fault that you were dealt a bad hand, but… it is your responsibility. How long will you allow your past to hold you back before you finally take control of your future?

Compared to the first, more nurturing voice in my head, this one was ice cold, and I did my best to tune it out.

The closer I got to Buffalo, the younger and more helpless I felt. When I was 150 miles away, I felt like I was sixteen years old. As I pulled off the highway and wound through the Buffalo city streets, I felt like I was eight, the same age I was when we packed all our belongings into garbage bags and walked out the door. Once I walked into the house, it was August 1983 all over again. The paint on the walls, the floors, the appliances and the furniture, all of it was the same. While it looked a lot smaller and out of date, it was still the haunted house I remembered, filled with years of grisly memories and palpable dark energy.

However, my father was warm and more affectionate than I remembered. Trunnis was always a charmer, and he acted genuinely happy to see me. As we caught up, I found myself laughing at his jokes, slightly confused by the man in front of me. After a while, he checked his watch and grabbed his coat.

He held the front door open for his wife, Sue, and me as we headed for the car.

"Where are we going?" I asked.

"You remember the schedule," he said. "It's time to open up."

The first thing I noticed about Skateland from the outside was that it needed a paint job. Inside, the floor and walls were chipped and stained, and the whole place smelled funky. The office had deteriorated too. That sofa we slept on as kids, where my mom caught him cheating on more than one occasion, still hadn't been replaced. It was filthy, and that's where I sat after the grand tour while my father headed upstairs to spin hip-hop records in the Vermillion Room.

I felt dizzy and disoriented. It was strange how far the old man had let his standards slip. He wasn't the strong, exacting, demanding figure I'd remembered. He was old, weak, soft in the middle, and lazy. He didn't even appear to be that mean anymore. He wasn't the Devil at all. He was human. Had I been feeding myself a false history? As I lingered in that office, steeped in the past, I wondered what else I'd been wrong about?

Then, at around ten o'clock, the bass line dropped upstairs and the ceiling started to shudder and shake. Within seconds, I heard hollering, laughter, and that steady stomping to the beat. In the same way a song can take you back to a distinct time and place, that thumping bass returned me to my darkest days. I'd been funneled into a relapse of my childhood nightmare.

I closed my eyes and saw myself as a first grader, tossing and turning on that very couch, trying to sleep after working all night and not being able to get more than a wink. My mother was there too, struggling to paper over our pain with "home-cooked" dinners prepared on portable electric burners in the cramped office. I saw the helplessness and fear in her eyes, and it brought back all the stress, pain, frustration, and depression that came with it. Those memories were real! There was no denying it!

I was disgusted to be sitting on that couch. I was sickened to have let my guard down and enjoyed my father's company, even for a few minutes. I felt like I was doing a disservice to my mother, and the longer I sat there and watched the ceiling shake, the more rage rose up inside until I was on my feet and racing up a back stairwell into the Vermillion Room, where my demon was slurping whiskey—the smoky elixir that gave him his power.

As a kid, I rarely saw the space in full bloom, and while it had lost most of its shine, it was still happening. What was once a glitzy nightclub serving funk to a well-dressed crowd had become a packed dive bar flush with hip-hop. Trunnis was in the DJ booth orchestrating the energy, spinning records, and sucking down scotch after scotch until closing time. I watched him work, drink, and flirt, and the more wasted he became, the more my memory synced with reality. After locking up, I drove us all to Denny's for an after-hours breakfast, just like old times. More than fifteen years had passed, yet the ritual remained the same as ever.

Trunnis was sloppy by then, and he could tell it made me uncomfortable, which ticked him off. While we waited for our food, he glared at me as he dissed my grandparents and claimed they were responsible for the breakup of his family. Liquor always brought his ugliness out, and I'd heard that argument so many times before, it didn't have much effect on me. But when he started in on my mom, I wasn't having any of it.

"Don't go there," I said quietly. But he didn't care. He barked about how everyone turned on him and how weak and sorry we all were. His spittle flew. The vein in his temple throbbed.

"Trunnis, please stop," Sue said. There was something in her tone, a mixture of fear and dread, that I recognized. She wasn't standing up and telling him how she felt. She was pleading with him. It reminded me so much of my mother and how powerless she felt when Trunnis would rage on and on. He was the type of guy who would call a woman over to the house at 3:55 p.m., knowing my mom would be coming home at four o'clock. He wanted her to catch them in the act to show her that he had all the power and would do whatever he wanted at any time of day or night. It's the same reason he beat me in front of her and did the same to her in front of me.

The very same day we left, Sue moved in, yet he often told her, and anyone else who would listen, how beautiful and smart my mother was, as if she were the one who got away. He needed Sue to feel she wasn't good enough for him, and never would be.

For the first time in my life, I felt for Sue and realized that Trunnis' specialty was the weaponization of disrespect. It was a tactic he used to bully women and children into submission. He knew that once he choked someone out mentally, they would lose all their fight and self-respect, which would make it easier to manipulate and dominate them. That's what he was after. Not love. He craved dominance and subservience. It was like oxygen to him. He harvested souls with violence and rage. He wanted the people closest to him to feel wounded and empty. Decades later, my mother still struggles with self-respect, decision-making, and confidence.

Trunnis' face was red from alcohol. His jaw clenched with tension as he kept talking trash. There was no doubt that he was the bully and abuser I remembered, but not because he hated my mom or Sue, or my brother or me, but because he was a sick, twisted old man who didn't believe he was worth anything and could not and would not help himself.

Years later, I would learn that he had suffered abuse when he was a kid. His father made him stand in front of a flaming-hot coal furnace in a dark room, and after a torturous waiting period, his dad would show up with a belt and lash him, buckle-side first. If he moved away from the belt, he'd get burned, so he had to accept his father's lashings and try not to move. He never dealt with his trauma, those memories festered into demons, and before he even knew it had happened, the victim became the abuser.

Whenever he got drunk and the party died down, he self-soothed by picking on people weaker than him. He beat them up. He ran them down. Sometimes, he threatened to kill them. But as soon as an abusive episode was over, he would erase it from history. The beatings we took never happened. He liked to think of himself as a big man but never accepted responsibility for anything he did that went wrong, which didn't make him any kind of a man at all. I suppose I was in that Denny's booth with him because part of me was hoping Trunnis would apologize, but he didn't think he had anything to be sorry for. He was straight-up delusional, and his delusions demoralized all of us. They were also contagious.

For years, he made me bleed, and he made me doubt myself. He transferred his demons to me through the lashes of his leather belt and the open palm of his hand, and like him, I grew up believing in delusions. I hadn't become an evil sociopath, but like him, I never took responsibility for my own shortcomings or my failures.

Sitting there listening to him rave made my blood run hot.

Sweat beaded on my forehead and all I could think about was payback. It was his turn to suffer at my hands. I wanted to make him bleed for my pain. I wanted to beat that man down right there in Denny's. I was hair-trigger close to allowing my father to turn me into a violent maniac just like I remembered him to be!

He recognized the fire in my eyes because it was as if he were looking into a mirror, and it scared him. The weather changed in our booth. He stopped ranting mid-sentence. His eyes went glassy and wide, and in the fluorescent light of the diner, he looked meek and small. I nodded as I recognized, in that very moment, the lie that inspired my trip to Buffalo.

I hadn't driven all the way from Indianapolis as some first step toward self-improvement. No, I was there looking for a free pass. I went to collect more evidence that all my many failures and disappointments stemmed from the same root cause: my father, Trunnis Goggins. I'd been hoping that everything I'd believed all those years was true because if Trunnis was indeed the Devil in disguise, that gave me someone to blame, and I was looking for a cop-out. I needed Trunnis to be the flaw in my existence in order to claim the lifetime warranty on my get-out-of-jail-free card.

Trunnis was flawed alright. He showed me that all over again. But he wasn't my flaw. The second voice was right. Unless I took responsibility for my demons, the ones he put on me, I had no shot at becoming anything other than a perpetual loser or another miserable hustler like him.

When the food arrived, Trunnis stuffed his face while I reflected on how much power I'd given him over the years. It wasn't his fault I experienced racism or barely graduated high school. Yes, he beat me and my brother up and tortured my mother. He was a sadistic man, but I hadn't lived with him since I was eight years old. When was I going to take my soul back from him? When was I going to own my own choices, my failures, my future? When would I finally accept responsibility for my life, take action, and wipe the slate clean?

Nobody said a word while I drove us back to Paradise Road. Trunnis watched me with a mix of drunken sadness, loss, and anger as I grabbed my car keys from the kitchen counter and walked straight out the door. I'd planned on spending the weekend, but I couldn't stand to be in his presence for one minute longer. While the words were never spoken, I believe we both knew that would be the last time we would ever see each other.

The funny thing was, I didn't even hate Trunnis anymore because I finally understood him. On the drive back home, I turned the volume way down on the nurturing voice in my head and tuned into reality. In place of excuses, it was time for ownership of exactly who I'd become in all of its ugliness, and that meant acknowledging that my thin skin was definitely part of the problem.

All of us are dealt circumstances in life we don't have any power to control. Sometimes, those things are painful; occasionally, they are tragic or inhuman. While the Accountability Mirror—which I tagged with sticky notes filled with real talk, daily tasks, and a few bigger goals—had helped me get to a certain point, those fixes were surface-level. I'd never attempted to dive down and solve the root cause of my problems, so I crumbled whenever life asked me to dig deeper and persevere in order to achieve something that could lead toward sustained success.

I'd spent my entire life in surface waters hoping that my luck would change and everything I'd dreamed of would fall into place for me. That night, on my drive home to Indiana, I accepted the hard truth that hoping and wishing are like gambling on long shots, and if I wanted to be better, I had to start living every day with a sense of urgency. Because that is the only way to turn the odds in your favor.

Reality can be brutal when all of your excuses are stripped away and you are exposed for exactly who and what you have become, but the truth can also be liberating. That night, I accepted the truth about myself. I finally swallowed reality, and now that I had, my future was undetermined. Anything was possible as long as I adopted a new mindset. I needed to become someone who refused to give in, who simply finds a way no matter what. I needed to become bulletproof, a living example of resilience.

Think of a packet of seeds scattered in a garden. Some seeds get more sunlight, more water, and are planted in nourishing topsoil, and because they are put in the right place at the right time, they can rise from seed to seedling to a thriving tree. Seeds planted in too much shade or that don't get enough water may never become anything at all unless someone transplants them—saves them—before it's too late.

Then there are those seedlings that look for the light on their own. They creep from the shade into the sunshine without being transplanted. They find it without anybody digging them up and placing them in the light. They find strength where there is none.

That is resilience.

Once we're born, our natural instinct is to look for ways to thrive. But not everybody does, and sometimes, there's a damn good reason for it. I was brought up in darkness. My roots were flimsy. I was barely tethered to rock-hard ground. My spirit, soul, and determination weren't nourished in the light, but on that ride home, I realized that only I have the power to determine my future, and I had a choice to make. I could continue living in the Haven of Low Expectations, where it was comfortable and safe to believe that my life was not my fault or my responsibility and that my dreams were just that—fantasies that would never be because time and opportunity were not and would never be on my side. Or I could leave all that behind for a world of possibility, much more pain, unfathomably hard work, and zero guarantees of success. I could choose resilience.

At twenty-four years old, a powerful force was gathering within me, waiting to be unleashed. I would soon call upon it to complete two Hell Weeks, become a member of the Navy Sea, Air, and Land (SEAL) Teams, and complete Army Ranger School. I'd compete in ultra races and break the world pull-up record. Thanks to that one night in Buffalo, New York, when I accepted my fate and became determined to tap into my resilience, I found the will to transform myself into the grittiest human being ever to find light where there was none.

I had never been a POW like John McCain and countless others, but I lived like a prisoner in my own mind for the first twenty-four years of my life. Once I'd liberated myself and begun to evolve, I learned that it is the rare warrior who embraces the adversity of being born into hell and then, with their own free will, chooses to add as much suffering as they can find to turn each day into a boot camp of resiliency. Those are the ones who don't stop at good enough. They aren't satisfied with just being better than they used to be. They are forever evolving and striving for the highest level of self. Eventually, I became one of them, which is why I was honored at the VFW Convention.

☙ ☙ ☙

"I'd like to thank my mom, who..." The audience gave me another round of applause as my sobs ebbed, and I returned to the present moment. "Who never picked me up when I fell. She let me pick myself up when I was knocked down."

By the time I was done speaking, all the emotion had drained clear. Honored and humbled to have received an award that most people would consider the crowning achievement of their career, I walked off that stage into the unknown. They say, "Iron sharpens iron," but I had left the military behind, and there was no one pushing me on a day-to-day basis any longer. *The hell with it.* I was always destined to be that one warrior. Content to be the one who sharpens his sword alone.

EVOLUTION NO. 1

I've worked in emergency medical services (EMS), on and off, for fifteen years. When an ambulance arrives on the scene of a severe trauma situation, we are immediately shotgunned into what's known as the "golden hour." In the vast majority of cases, sixty minutes is all the time we have to save a critically injured victim. The clock starts the moment the accident happens and doesn't stop until the patient arrives at a hospital trauma center. By the time we get to the scene of the accident, we are already behind, which means it is vital that our assessment of each patient is rapid and on point.

Some are identified as "Load and Go" because they need specific, time-sensitive interventions that we can't do ourselves. Others are identified as "Stay and Play." Though their condition may be dire, they have issues our skills are built to address to ensure they survive the trip to the hospital. One of the first things we do when we get to a patient is check their ABCs:

airway, breathing, and circulation. We need to make sure their airway is unobstructed, their lungs are inflating, and they aren't bleeding profusely. Usually, ABC issues are obvious, but every once in a while, we come across a distracting injury.

Picture a shattered leg twisted way up over the victim's head. When you see a limb in a place it does not belong, it's easy to become fixated. It looks so gruesome that human instinct is to address that problem first and block everything else out. I've seen a lot of EMS personnel get sucked down that rabbit hole, but a badly broken and dislocated leg typically won't kill anyone, unless it distracts us from realizing that their airway is also blocked or that they are gurgling because their lungs are filled with fluid and they are in danger of bleeding out internally. A distracting injury, in the EMS universe, is anything that entices a medical professional to forget their procedures. It can happen to anyone, which is why we are trained to remain alert to those distractions. It truly is a matter of life or death.

The same can be said of the distracting injuries I carried. By the time I turned twenty-four, I was too distracted by child abuse, neglect, and racist taunts to see all of the messed-up things in my life over which I had direct influence. Nothing that happened to me could be considered a fatal condition on its own, yet I spent so much time worrying about what my father did to us, and felt so alone, I was refusing to live. And when you spend your life regretting what was or asking, "Why me?" you eventually die having accomplished nothing at all.

The trip to Buffalo was pure distraction. I wasn't ready to put in the work to change my life, so I went on an evidence-collecting mission. In fact, by the time I figured it out, it was almost impossible for me to become a SEAL. I was so heavy that if I had been even a few pounds heavier, I would not have been able to lose the necessary weight in the allotted time. I had to take extreme measures—like eating two tiny meals while working out six to eight hours a day for ten weeks—but when I started to shed weight and shift my mindset, I realized I had never been as alone as I'd thought. I'd always told myself that nobody could possibly understand me or what I went through, but as I looked around, I noticed that there were a lot of people out there with distracting injuries stuck neck-deep in their past. These days, I hear from them all the time.

Some suffered child abuse or lost a parent very young. Others grew up feeling ugly or stupid. They were bullied and beaten down or had no friends in school at all. It's not always the childhood minefield that screws us up. There is no shortage of psychological and emotional snags in adult life. Every day, people suffer bankruptcy, foreclosure, divorce, and catastrophic injury. They get cheated or robbed by their so-called loved ones. They get sexually assaulted. They lose everything they own in a fire or flood. Their children die.

It's so easy to get lost in the fog of life. Tragedy hunts us all, and any event that causes suffering will linger longer than it should if you let it. Because our sad stories enable us to grade ourselves on a forgiving curve. They give us latitude and justification to stay lazy, weak-minded people, and the longer it takes for us to process that pain, the harder it is to reclaim our lives.

Sometimes, weakness and laziness are rooted in hate and anger, and until we receive the confession, apology, or compensation we believe we are owed, we stay stuck in our self-pity as a form of self-righteous rebellion against our tormentors or even against life itself. Some of us become entitled. We think our pain entitles us to feel sorry for ourselves or that we are entitled to good fortune because we've survived so much. Of course, feeling entitled doesn't make it so. Understand, the clock is always ticking, and at some point, your golden hour will expire unless you take action.

People who get lost in their past, the ones who bore their friends and family with the same tragic story over and over without showing a hint of progress, remind me of a skydiver who becomes too fixated on their tangled parachute. They know they have a backup ready to go but burn so much time trying to fix the primary chute that they forget to track their altimeter, and by the time they cut the first chute away and pull the second ripcord, it's too late. Part of the problem is that they have become terrified of pulling that second cord because if it's also compromised, then they truly will be helpless. That is a mental trap set by fear. We cannot afford to remain afraid of cutting away dead weight to save ourselves.

I was that skydiver for far too long. My father was violent. My mom was broken. I was bullied, laughed at, and misunderstood. Check, check, and checkmate. And yet, I was breathing free, and I was not bleeding. Physically, I was alive and well and perfectly capable of cutting all of that garbage away. I'd wasted way too much of my life telling myself the same sad story. I needed to move forward. It was time to write something new.

If an act of God or nature tore your life apart, the good news is that you really have nobody to blame. Yet, the randomness of it all can feel so personal, as if you've been marked for doom by the fates. If you feel wronged by somebody else, you may be waiting on a confession or an apology in order to move forward, but I'm sorry to say the apology—that tearful confession you've been dreaming of—will never come. The good news is you don't need anybody else to free you from your trauma. You can do it on your own.

My father never apologized to me. Nobody ever said sorry for anything I went through. I had to come to the conclusion that while I didn't deserve any of it, I was my main problem and primary obstacle. I'd given Trunnis Goggins all of my power. I had to take it back. I had to diffuse my demon. I had to shrink him down to the lowly, pathetic figure he was by humanizing him. Just as there was no other way to come out of the gauntlet that was my childhood except screwed up, I had to see that he was a mortally flawed piece of crap because of what he went through. Once I understood that, it was up to me to either do the hard work to break that cycle or stay cursed.

Like medics on the scene of a car accident, we all must act with a sense of urgency and tune into that ticking clock in the back of our minds. Because there is a drop-dead time on everything we do in life. All our dreams and visions come with expiration dates etched in invisible ink. Windows of opportunity can and do close, so it is imperative that we do not waste time on foolishness. None of us have any clue what's coming for us or when our time might run out, which is why I do my best to ignore anything that is counterproductive. I'm not suggesting we act like robots, but we need to understand that forward motion gives our lives momentum. We need to remember that sometimes chaos will descend and a clear highway can be wiped out by a flash flood in the blink of an eye.

When that happens, a lot of people look for a cozy place to hunker down and hide out until the storm passes. "I'm only human," they say. When chaos rains down upon them and they feel drained and powerless, they cannot conceive of a way to keep going. I understand that impulse, but if I had succumbed to the "I'm only human" mentality, I never would have dug myself out of the deep hole I was in at twenty-four years old.

Because the second you utter those words, the white towel is fluttering in the air, and your mind stops looking for more fuel. I didn't know for sure if I'd ever find my way out of the darkness. I just knew that I could not throw in the towel, and neither can you. Because there is no towel in our corner. There is only water and a cut man. And if those are your only options, you have no choice but to keep fighting until you overcome every last thing that once held you back.

> You have been preoccupied for way too long. It's time to switch your focus to the things that will slingshot you forward. #DistractingInjuries #NeverFinished

CHAPTER TWO

MERRY CHRISTMAS

On the day after Christmas 2018, Kish and I had breakfast with my brother, Trunnis Jr., my mother, and my niece Alexis at the aptly named Loveless Café in Nashville. It was the perfect place for a Goggins family breakfast, considering our history with the so-called happiest time of the year. Growing up, my friends made such a big deal about Christmas. They talked about it and their wish lists for weeks ahead of time. They watched the same old Christmas movies and sang the same corny songs. To me, it was just another day on the calendar, no different than the rest, because of how I came up.

In Buffalo, Christmas was a marketing opportunity for my father. While most kids were playing with their new toys and slipping into fresh gear, we were scraping gum off the skating-rink floors, then polishing them and prepping the building for an all-night skate. Once we escaped to Indiana, my mom was so shell-shocked that she couldn't have cared less about any holidays. Consumed with finding work, a place to live, and having a social life of her own, Christmas—and my experience of it—did not register on her priority list.

It had been three years since I'd last seen and communicated with my brother, in the days after his eldest daughter was killed. We've always had an awkward relationship because our perspectives on our childhood are so different. When my dad was abusing us, my brother always attempted to be a peacemaker, and that required him to make excuses for our father no matter how vicious he was. He wanted everything to be kumbaya. When our dad came after our mother, Trunnis Jr. made it a point to escape to his room, while I made sure to watch. I saw things as they really were, and that made me a fighter. Trunnis Jr. remembers things as he wished they had been. I've never blamed him for it. We were all doing our best to survive somehow. My mom couldn't protect either of us. She was beaten just as badly as we were. It was as if there were four different versions of the same reality show streaming from the same house all at once. The dissonance was impossible not to feel and absorb.

When I was nine years old, my brother chose to leave us and our new life in Indiana to live with our father, and we were never close after that. However, he will always be my only brother, so when I heard Kayla had been killed, I dropped everything to be with him. I will always care about him, and I admire him for surviving our childhood to become an amazing father and earn his PhD. Still, we share too much history and experienced it too differently for it to be anything but awkward when we get together. So, when he told me what he had planned after breakfast, I wasn't the least bit surprised.

"We're driving to Buffalo," he said with a grin, "to show the kids around and pay our respects to the old man." I glanced at my mother, who would be accompanying him and his family on their trip down memory lane. She couldn't look me in the eye. Although she and I don't always remember every little thing the same way either, we know we survived hell. Like any good revisionist historian, Trunnis Jr. is still trying to convince himself otherwise. Which is why Buffalo remains his favorite city. He makes the trip as often as possible, and whenever he does, he visits the grave of our tormentor.

For survivors of trauma, denial is a tantalizing numbing agent. It allows you to rewrite your past and sell yourself some fiction. In my brother's tale, Buffalo was a happy place, and our father was a pillar of the community. When we were kids, he forgave our father quicker than a priest in a confessional, and as an adult, his selective memory gives his childhood a brighter sheen, which makes him feel less damaged. But whether he wants to acknowledge it or not, damage was done. If he had experienced things the way my mom and I had, he wouldn't subject her to a stroll through his personal fantasyland, as if Buffalo weren't the torture chamber she'd had to escape many years ago.

By 2018, I'd mastered my childhood demons. I was the puppeteer, and all the skeletons in my closet were on strings I controlled. My mother didn't deny what had happened to us either, but like my brother, she preferred to avoid her pain. She hated discussing her experience with my father or even thinking about it, and later, when she described that trip back to Buffalo with Trunnis Jr., she said that she'd felt dazed. Everything looked unfamiliar. Even the house on Paradise Road. She didn't recognize a single building or street name. It was as if her memory had been wiped like a hard drive, and she was seeing it all—the house, Skateland, all of her old familiar haunts—for the first time.

Trauma will do that. It redacts places, names, and incidents if you don't do the hard work to process the difficult times. If, like my brother, you stash it away in the way back of your mind—deep enough that it becomes impossible to reach—or, like my mom, try to ignore it because it's too much to confront, one day, it won't just be the bad memories that are repressed. Entire chunks of your life will have slipped through your fingers.

My mother could have gone to Buffalo with a game plan. It should have been her victory lap. When we left, Trunnis told her that she'd become a prostitute and I'd become a gangster. Instead, she became a Senior Associate Vice President at a medical college in Nashville making six figures. Trunnis Jr. is a college professor and family man. I'm a Retired Navy SEAL who had just been honored by the VFW and was the author of a new book. But she didn't go to Trunnis' grave to tell him any of that. She floated above the moment in a bubble she'd built to survive another weekend in Buffalo, New York. Like most of us, she didn't want to feel her pain, so she failed to find the power in it.

A lot of us are trapped in our own brains, shackled by long-gone demons who might even be dead. We refuse to discuss or acknowledge what happened, so when we overcome it all, we fail to recognize it or even feel it. My mom left Buffalo a shell of herself and became a successful, professional woman, but she was still cowering before the demon that stole her soul. She should have written Trunnis a letter telling him what he'd missed and who he'd unleashed. She should have read it out loud to him at his grave. Not so he knew what she'd become, but so she knew it! She needed to take her soul back and introduce herself to herself!

Denial is self-protecting, but it's also self-limiting. Accepting your full truth, including all your faults, imperfections, and missteps, allows you to evolve, expand your possibilities, seek redemption, and explore your true potential. And until you unpack your baggage, it will be impossible to know what your potential really is. The whole truth can't haunt you if it serves you.

Kish and I were scheduled to fly to Florida that night to celebrate a belated Christmas with her tight-knit family. Christmas had always been a big deal to Kish, and though a cozy holiday house sounded soft as hell to me, she's the greatest woman I've ever met. We'd become partners in life and in business, and I wanted her to be happy. If that meant a trip to Norman Rockwell's Florida Christmas, so be it. But there weren't gonna be any matching pajama pictures, I promise you that!

We had several hours before the flight, and Kish spent them digging into the sales numbers for my first book, *Can't Hurt Me*. It had been out for less than a month and already sold more copies than I ever imagined possible. After more than five years and multiple setbacks, the book I'd envisioned was finally out in the world, and it was a hit.

While some people may not be surprised by the book's success, there are countless others who most definitely are. Prior iterations of the book proposal had been passed on and turned down by numerous publishing houses that didn't see the value in my story. Case in point: in 2016, I presented a one-hundred-plus-page book proposal to Ed Victor. He was a legend in the literary world and was introduced to me by none other than Marcus Luttrell, who had worked with him on his bestselling book *Lone Survivor*. Ed also repped rock stars, like Eric Clapton and Keith Richards, and some of the biggest novelists in the game. He was once quoted as having grown up "...perceiving life as a long highway littered with green lights." In a different article, he mentioned that the criteria he used to determine the publishing potential of a given project boiled down to three questions. "Is the person fabulous? Is the work good? And is there a lot of money in it?" My book proposal did not pass that particular evaluation. But I give him credit. He didn't sugarcoat the bad news in his rejection email.

From: Ed Victor
Date: June 27, 2016, 6:46:16 AM PDT
To: David
Cc: Jennifer Kish
Subject: Your book

Dear David

I said I would get back to you on Monday, so here I am...but you are not going to like what I have to say.

...my assessment of its value—and its sales potential—are in no way aligned with yours. I could be wrong—I certainly have been in the past!—but I don't see this as a book that will command a big advance and sell large amounts of copies...

When I told you I would be honest in my reaction to this project, you warned me that, if I said No, I'd then see it high up on the NY Times Bestseller List and deeply regret my decision. You may well be right, but because my assessment of the value and commercial prospects of the book are so far below yours, I would not be the right agent for it. You need someone with 101% enthusiasm who will go out and prove me hopelessly wrong (not for the first time).

...

All best
Ed

PS I will tell Marcus about my decision, since it was he who tried to bring us together.

It shouldn't have surprised me that the guy who grew up with nothing but green lights couldn't relate to a life stifled by red lights, potholes, and stop signs, but he was the industry expert and didn't see my story as accessible. That was a problem, and it was discouraging in the moment, but it didn't make me angry, and I never second-guessed my own value. I knew that my life, my story, and my approach were non-traditional. Their cookie cutter didn't work on me. I couldn't be boxed and packaged to industry standards. Roger that. When had I ever been the perfect fit for anything at all? Never. But I still managed to find success.

What Ed Victor saw as a disadvantage—the fact that I couldn't be easily defined and sold—was actually my greatest asset. My approach, background, and accomplishments all proved one thing: I am the ultimate underdog. That's been the truth my whole life, and if no one could see my potential, it would be up to me to show them what they missed.

There are libraries packed with books on how to be happy and the power of positivity, but nobody prepares you for the dark ages, and the power of my story was in my grind through tough times to become the one person inspiring you to never be satisfied. Ed and all the other industry experts I'd met weren't interested in that because they didn't get it. That didn't mean that the book wouldn't sell. It just meant I had to double down on what made me unique, maintain faith in myself and my vision, and work harder.

In 2017, I signed with a new literary agent and put together another proposal that earned me a $300,000 advance from a major publishing house. That's good money, but while I waited for the contract to come through, I became conflicted. Was I ready to sell my story to someone else? Did I want or even need an editor to help me tell it?

I was the only one who knew how much blood I'd shed and how many times I'd been baptized in sweat to get me to this point. There were too many all-nighters and pre-dawn wake-up calls to count. I'd been knocked down hundreds of times. I'd pushed my mind, body, and soul to the very edge. Like Andy Dufresne in *Shawshank Redemption*, I'd spent more than twenty years scraping away at the prison wall of my mind with a blunt hammer, and I needed the final say when it came to the edits and who made money off of my story. After many days and nights of turning it over in my head, I realized the only way to ensure that was to publish the book myself.

Once I killed the deal, my agent cussed me out. He told me I was off his client roster and that I would be lucky to sell ten thousand copies. Basically, he said, "Merry Christmas, Goggins," and cut me loose. He wasn't alone. Almost everybody I turned to for advice—people who knew how the industry worked and what it took to succeed—said I was a fool.

So be it.

You cannot be afraid to disappoint people. You have to live the life you want to live. Sometimes, that means being the person who can stand alone in a crowded room and be totally comfortable with that.

Now, does that mean you won't be nervous or that it will all go smoothly? Hell no. When you're on the ramp of a C-130 at twenty thousand feet, it's okay if your knees start to buckle because you know time is short and freefall is imminent, but the second you leap from the aircraft, you must commit to the jump. If you don't, you will flop around, dangerously out of control, and fall too fast. You need to commit in order to focus on keeping a stable body position. And never look down. Focus on the horizon. That is your perspective. That is your future.

Instead of receiving a big advance, I spent 90 percent of my life savings—more than the advance I would have received—to put out a book of the same quality as anything the major publishers release, and I produced my own audiobook with an entirely new spin. It was risky, but trailblazers never take the smooth roads thousands of others have already traveled. They go cross-country and dig their own path forward. I'd been outside the box my whole life. I'd been smashing cookie cutters for nearly two decades, and this was the biggest bet I'd ever made on myself.

"You're on the *New York Times* Best Seller list," Kish said. She looked up from her laptop and flashed a smile. She was proud, and I was too. Not because I cared about the *New York Times* Best Seller list, or even that it was selling at all, but because I knew the book was an honest reflection of my life and all I put into it. And, admittedly, after being told that making any best seller list was "absolutely not going to happen" and "impossible" for a self-published book by a first-time author, it was satisfying to defy the odds one more time.

I was borderline illiterate in fifth grade. That night, I imagined sitting down with that eleven-year-old kid who struggled so much in class and was so hungry for acceptance. If I told him that one day he would become a bestselling author, he'd have laughed in my face.

I shook my head, chuckled to myself, and swallowed a handful of vitamins. Without warning, my heart began to race. I put two fingers to my carotid and checked my watch. My pulse shot from a steady fifty beats per minute to 150 beats per minute and back again without any set rhythm.

As an EMT and someone who had recovered from multiple heart surgeries, I knew right away that I was in atrial fibrillation, or AFib, which is when the upper chambers of the heart, the atria, are out of rhythm with the lower chambers, the ventricles. I'd experienced a similar episode nine years earlier after my first heart surgery when one of the patches failed. Did another patch fail, or was this something new?

I didn't tell Kish right away. She'd worked for months without a break to help turn *Can't Hurt Me* into a hit, and she couldn't wait to go home and be with her family. Instead, I tried to control my heart rate through vagal maneuvers, like equalizing the pressure in my sinuses with the Valsalva technique and squeezing my knees into my chest, forcing a gag or a cough, and massaging the carotid sinus. Those techniques had been proven to reset the pressure in the body and click the heart back into rhythm. Deep breathing can help too, but nothing worked, and the longer it went on, the dizzier I became and the graver the danger.

AFib can turn blood clots into embolisms that block blood vessels in the brain or heart, causing strokes and heart failure. People with sickle cell trait, like me, are at a higher risk for blood clots. Hours passed. I pretended everything was cool while my pulse sketched a dire electrocardiogram in my mind's eye, but when Kish zipped her suitcase and turned to me, ready to roll to Florida, she could see something was very wrong. We weren't headed to the airport. We were going to the emergency room.

The day after Christmas is dead in most public places, but holiday season in the ER is always bumping. Maybe it's the alcohol, the family strife, the loneliness, or a combination of all three. When I was fourteen years old, my mother's fiancé, Wilmoth, was shot and killed the day after Christmas, which is why whenever the calendar leans into late December, I think more about trauma than Santa.

The ER was packed when we walked through the sliding glass doors. I slumped into one of the few spare seats in the waiting room, dizzy as hell. Medics, doctors, and nurses blurred as they hustled between treatment areas, wheeling patients around the squeaky tiled floors on gurneys and in wobbly old wheelchairs. The PA system crackled. Fluorescent lights buzzed overhead. Kish sat beside me and filled out paperwork as I closed my eyes and took yet another deep breath.

Minutes later, or maybe it was hours, I did the same thing in front of a young doctor in a curtained-off treatment area. He wasn't a cardiologist, and when I explained I'd had two heart surgeries, he took the news a bit too casually. He listened to my heartbeat, tagged me up with sensors, and watched my pulse scratch out a rhythm on his ECG monitor. Then, he told me what I'd just told him.

"You're in AFib."

"Roger that." I shot him some side eye. Kish caught it.

"What can you do for him, doctor?" she asked.

"We're going to put you on a drip and see how you respond."

A nurse came in and tapped my vein, and the meds seemed to work. Within minutes, my pulse relaxed and my dizziness eased, but when the doc strolled back in an hour later, he looked confused as he read the monitors.

"Well, your pulse has calmed down, but you're still in AFib," he said. "I'm going to call a cardiologist upstairs and see what we can do here."

I didn't need to hear what the cardiologist had to say to know my fate. I'd studied AFib cases, and if breathing techniques, equalization, and meds don't sync the chambers, the next step is to shock the heart, to restart it like you would a frozen computer. I'd seen videos of it, and I was terrified.

It's funny, my two heart surgeries never scared me. I knew death was a risk with both of them, but my mortality didn't register at all back then, and I greeted them with a shoulder shrug. That night in Nashville, I felt differently about life and death.

Can't Hurt Me had changed me, and my latest metamorphosis ran much deeper than commercial success and the public's enthusiasm for my story. Writing that book allowed me to process the horror I'd gone through one last time, and publishing it myself gave me a clean slate. People had always assumed a lot of things about me. *Can't Hurt Me* finally allowed me to speak my truth, and I felt vindicated. I could finally be at peace with my life and all that I put into it and accomplished. Then, right on cue, my heart skipped like a scratched record and there I was, back in life's crosshairs.

Merry Christmas, indeed!

While Kish called her parents and wiped away tears, I confronted a bitter possibility. I believed my role on this earth was to suffer and overcome so I could teach others how to do the same, but now that that period of my life appeared to be over, I had to wonder: was I suddenly expendable? My self-talk flip-flopped between feeling sorry for myself and being royally pissed. My anxiety was off the charts. I was not sneering at death like back in the day. I was afraid. Desperate for more life.

A technician arrived and shaved my chest. She put one electrode on my chest and another on my back. Then, the doctor strolled in and asked Kish to grab a seat in the waiting room out front. He read the monitors, glanced over at me, and hit the switch. Two hundred joules flowed through me, and everything went blank. For a fraction of a second, I was suspended between heartbeats. He hit me again, and I screamed as I came to. Kish heard me take the Lord's name in vain all the way in the waiting room, something I never do. That's how much it hurt. But it worked. I was synced.

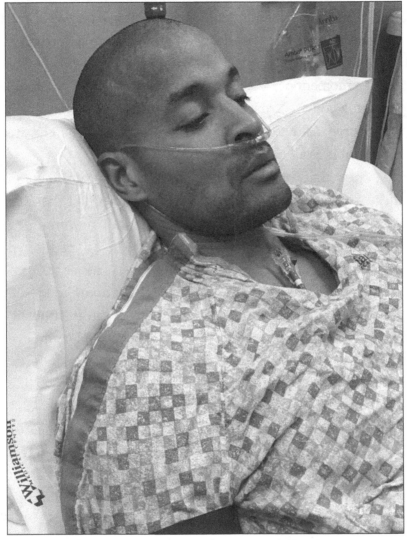

Trying to control the fear of being shocked

The doctor sent me home with a normal pulse, a battery of tests to be scheduled to make sure there was nothing structurally wrong with my heart, and a tweaked-out soul. This is how life works. One second, you are talking about the *New York Times* Best Seller list, and the next, you run the risk of not being able to live to see tomorrow. It literally happens that quickly.

Nothing is permanent. Life is the ultimate competitor. It takes no days off, and it won't care if you've made some money or got a promotion at work. All that means is you are good to go for a moment or two. No matter how tough and successful you think you are, trust me, there is a semi coming around a blind curve, ready to smack you in the mouth when you are comfortable as all hell.

I knew that, but I also thought my heart issues were in the rearview mirror. Now, I could see how ridiculous that was. When you are always in the grind, you think there will come a time when the rough road, blitzed with potholes and littered with blown tires, will smooth out, but that is never the case. In fact, if you go through life expecting that smooth road, you won't be prepared when a pothole opens up on freshly laid blacktop and rocks you sideways one warm and pleasant evening. That's what Merry Christmas means in Gogglish. It has nothing to do with the holiday. It's about the surprise "gifts" life has wrapped up, just waiting for you to stumble into.

Which is another way of saying I lost something essential in that emergency room. As dawn broke on the drive home, I felt like Samson running around bald in the hamster wheel of my mind. I didn't know who I was anymore. Was I still a savage, or was I just another squawking head?

Some people might be put off by the term, but to me, calling someone a "savage" is the highest compliment. A savage is an individual who defies odds, who has a will that cannot be tamed, and who, when knocked down, will always get back up!

If the doctors told me that I had to stop running and working out hard in the gym, I would cancel everything. I'd pull the plug on all future speaking engagements and on my social media channels. I've always been a man of action and service, and I know I would not be able to inspire people by simply talking about the things I did in my past. I gave myself one rule before joining social media: if I can't live it, I won't speak it. Before I bedded down that night, I decided that if my body wouldn't cooperate anymore, *Can't Hurt Me* would be my swan song, and I would disappear.

EVOLUTION NO. 2

Never waste a single thing. It was a lesson I first learned in Brazil, Indiana, when a classmate brought me a gift after school. I didn't get a lot of presents growing up, so when he handed me that one, I was a thirsty little kid. I wanted to tear that package open and see what I got. The first loud rip got my grandfather's attention. He poked his head into the room and surveyed the scene. "Calm down," he said. Then, he handed me a pair of scissors. "That's good wrapping paper. We can reuse that."

A lot of us grew up with grandparents seasoned by the Great Depression, who knew we were working with finite resources. Even those who made a nice living didn't take comfort or plenty for granted, and I guess that rubbed off on me. To this day, I abhor waste. I eat all my leftovers, and when my tube of toothpaste flattens out, I don't just roll it up to squeeze out the remainder, I cut that tube open and put it in a Ziploc baggie until I've used every last drop.

Everything must be utilized. Especially the energy in volatile, potentially damaging emotions like fear and hate. You have to learn how to handle them—how to mine them—and once you master that craft, any negative emotion or event that bubbles up in your brain or gets lobbed your way, like a grenade, can be used as fuel to make you better. But to get there, you must literally listen to yourself.

In 2009, I was training to ride in a three-thousand-mile cycling race called the Race Across America, better known as RAAM. I was still full-time in the military, so I had to wake up extra early to fit in my fifty- to one hundred-mile rides before work. My weekend training rides stretched out over two hundred miles—sometimes I rode upwards of five hundred miles—often on the narrow shoulders of busy highways. I did all that because the RAAM's distance scared me. The monotony of being able to stay locked in on a bicycle for days at a time without sleep freaked me out. The race burrowed so deep into my psyche that I wasn't sleeping well. To demystify the experience, I made a point of chronicling each ride on a handheld tape recorder. I described everything I saw and felt in granular detail.

It was mostly just me on a bike with cars, Harleys, and semis zooming past. I smelled all the exhaust, felt the wind slap me upside the head, and tasted the grit of the open road. When I veered onto the blue roads, I wouldn't see a single car for fifty miles, but that white line was ever-present. Whether the shoulder was wide, thin, or nonexistent, the white line was always there.

I listened to those tapes at night and visualized the white line a thousand times. I became entranced by the simplicity of it, which helped minimize everything else about the race. And though I didn't enter RAAM that year because of emergency heart surgery, I knew I'd stumbled onto a system to minimize my fears and build confidence that I'd use for years to come.

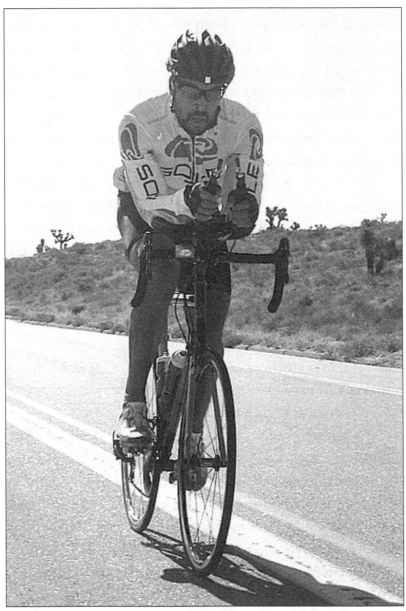

I can't possibly fathom the hours spent alone riding the white line

When I started speaking to Fortune 500 companies and professional ballclubs for a living, I had to be willing to reveal my brutal life story to successful people—including millionaires and billionaires who had heard it all. This wasn't some simple recruiting trip to a high school where students were easily impressed, and all my anxiety around public speaking resurfaced. Once again, I broke out the tape recorder. I spoke my fears and my trauma—which not that many people knew about—into that microphone and discovered a strange, unexpected alchemy. My fear and trauma were transformed into energy and confidence.

Many people write out their darkest moments in a journal or diary and hope to gain some leverage on whatever it is they survived or are struggling to overcome. I've kept a journal for years, but there are levels to this, and a written archive is the entry level. Audio recordings are more interactive and accessible and have a more profound effect on the mind.

If you were bullied, abused, or sexually assaulted and are willing to speak the unfiltered truth into the microphone and listen to it over and over, after a period of time, it will become just another story. A powerful story, for sure, but the poison will be neutralized, and the power will be yours.

This is not a task to take lightly. If you've survived acute trauma, you don't want to think about what you were doing on the day it happened, what you heard and how you felt, or how your life capsized afterward. Do it anyway. The more color and context you can add to the track, the sooner you will walk the streets with your headphones on and your head held high. When people see you coming, they might think you're listening to an Eminem jam. But no, it's your deepest trauma, the scene of your supposed destruction, on repeat. With each subsequent listen, you will claim more and more power and gain enough transformational energy to change your life.

Most people don't even want to think about their darkest moments, much less talk about it. They refuse to speculate in the harsh wilderness of their past because they are afraid of exposure. Believe me, there's gold in them there hills. I know because I was the Black dude in the cowboy hat, hip deep in the icy stream panning for nuggets. And if you find the courage to paint the picture of your worst nightmare in the spoken word, then listen to it until it soaks in and saturates your mind, until you can hear it without any emotional reaction or spillover, it will no longer make you cower or cry. It will make you strong. Strong enough to walk out on stage and tell the whole world what they did to you, and how it didn't break you. It made you powerful.

Recording yourself isn't just a reliable tool for neutralizing trauma. It can change the dynamic of almost any situation or mood. If you use it properly, it can also keep you honest. One day a couple of years ago, not long after ramping up my training from ten miles of running per day to twenty or more, I felt drained and sore, too tired to run, and kept telling myself that I needed a day off. As I relaxed on the couch, I tuned into my self-talk. Then, I grabbed my recorder and whined into the microphone. I wanted to hear how it sounded out loud. I was real with myself. I cataloged my recent runs and nagging injuries and described how I thought a day off might help me. I made a solid case for a much-needed rest day, but when I played it back, the jury of one was unconvinced. Because my inner crybaby was suddenly the emperor with no clothes. Buck naked in the light of day, he was impossible to ignore and even harder to stomach. I was off the couch and out on the road in a matter of seconds.

Many people wake up with dread or doubt day after day. They dread their workouts, their class load, or their job. Maybe they have a test or presentation that makes them nervous, or they know that the day's workout will hurt. While they linger in bed, they tune into their soft, forgiving self-talk, which doesn't make it any easier to get up and moving. Most people rise up eventually, but they remain in a daze for hours because they aren't fully engaged with their lives. Their self-talk has made them numb to the moment, and they sleepwalk through half the day before they finally perk up.

The way we speak to ourselves in moments of doubt is crucial, whether or not the stakes are high. Because our words become actions, and our actions build habits that can coat our minds and bodies with the plaque of ambivalence, hesitancy, and passivity and separate us from our own lives. If any of this sounds familiar, grab your phone and record your inner dialogue as soon as you wake up. Don't hold back. Spill all your dread, laziness, and stress into the mic. Now listen to it. Nine times out of ten, you won't like what you hear. It will make you cringe. You wouldn't want your girlfriend or boyfriend, your boss, or your kids to hear your unfiltered weakness. But you should.

Because then you can repurpose it. You can use it to remind yourself that changes must be made. Listening might inspire you to commit to your life in a deeper way, to be your best at work, at school, or in the gym. It can challenge you to rewrite the narrative so that when you bed down, you won't feel like you wasted another valuable day.

Do it again the next morning, but this time, once you get through listening to all your whining about what you don't want to do, sit up in bed and lay down a second take. Pretend you're motivating a friend or loved one who is going through challenges. Be respectful of the issues they face, but be positive, forceful, and realistic too. This is a skill that demands repetition, and if you do it regularly, you'll find that it won't take long for your self-talk to flip from doubt and dread to optimism and empowerment. The conditions of your life might not change a whole lot at first, but your words will make sure that your approach does change, and that will eventually enable you to shift everything. But you must speak the truth and be willing to listen to it. Don't be afraid of your weakness or doubt. Don't be embarrassed and pretend it doesn't exist. It surfaced for a reason, so use it to flip the dynamic of your life.

Lately, I've used this technique with the hate that comes at me online. Most people in my position don't read negative comments or emails. They have someone else screen and then erase them. I see hate as just another fuel source. I see the beauty and power in it, and I never let it go to waste. When the negative comments come in, and they always do, I capture them in a screenshot and speak them into my microphone. In 2021, I posted an image of my swollen left knee, which inspired a flood of negative comments. Some claimed to have seen my breakdown coming and counted it as a personal win. Others simply liked seeing me in pain.

"I'm tired of hearing you run your mouth," one of them wrote.

"I hope I never see your Black butt run again," wrote another.

They were trying to salt my wounds. They wanted me to feel the sting, which I did, and hoped it would bring me down even further. It didn't. I loved those comments. I loved them so much I made a mixtape. I printed them all out, recorded myself saying each one, and then I looped it. Whenever I have a bad day, I listen to it. Sometimes, I walk around the house savoring it in full stereo.

Most people only mine the positive stuff. They want everything and everyone to be nice and hunky-dory. They get filled up on sweetness and recoil from the dark, bitter pill of hate. But there's not nearly as much fuel in atta' boys and accolades as there is in hate. Luckily, the world is filled with jealous, insecure haters. If you don't get negative comments on social media, find your fuel in the thoughtless comment of a friend or the doubt of a teacher or coach. I'm sure it stings when you feel slighted, underestimated, criticized, or excluded. Just know that the heat you feel is free energy waiting to be burned. Don't crawl up in a corner worried about the people who disrespect you. Repackage what you're hearing and feeling until it works for you!

That is a winner's mentality. Winners in life see everything they experience and everything they hear, see, and feel as pure energy. They train their minds to find it. They drop into the gnarly crevices to mine golden nuggets of trauma, doubt, and hate. They do not live disposable, single-use lives. They discard nothing and refurbish everything. They find strength in the bullying and heartbreak, in their defeats and failures. They harvest it from the people who hate them personally and from the online trolls too.

Some people go to sleep with a meditation app. Others open the windows to the night sounds or stream white noise, whale songs, or the lullaby of the sea lapping some lonely shore. When I bed down at night, I listen to my haters. And it's obvious those weak cowards don't have the slightest idea who they are dealing with.

I'm the person who turns their every negative word into my positive progress. I take what they serve me, roll it up in that wrapping paper I saved way back when, and give it right back to them in the form of another work-out, another long run, and another year of leveling up. Honestly, I should thank them. They make me stronger and more determined to achieve my goals. Which only makes them hate me even more.

It's time to make your own mixtape. #TapeRecordYourself #NeverFinished

CHAPTER THREE

THE MENTAL LAB

Five weeks after Christmas, it had become obvious that my whole life had changed. The unexpected attention and notoriety that came with and followed the release of *Can't Hurt Me* was as humbling as it was disorienting. After decades of grinding in the shadows outside the public eye, I was now spotlit.

I'd always felt most at home in the margins. During my military career, I'd go on my longest runs and rucks before anyone else woke up. While others were relaxing or partying after a hard day or week of work, I stayed in to study my dive tables, pack and repack my parachute, or run and grind in the gym deep into the night. Everything I did on my own time was for my own personal fulfillment and growth. I sure didn't do it for attention. Yet, I was often misunderstood.

I was carrying a boulder as big as the world on my back, just trying to get to the other side of the darkness that was chasing me down. I was terrified that if I stopped getting better, if I gave myself a break from any of it, all my insecurities and innate laziness would get the drop on me again. Anytime I felt physically exhausted or mentally zapped, I pictured my twenty-four-year-old fat self glaring at me with a big smile on his face. A smile that said, *"I'm still here, loser. I am who you really are, and I'm not going anywhere."*

I looked at each day as an opportunity to mine the negativity that had colonized my brain and became fascinated by the power of the mind and how it can work for us and against us. Often, it falls prey to the merry-go-round of emotions and situational conditions that cause confusion and sap us of focus, force, and fortitude, all of which have a natural tendency to ebb and flow like the tide. My early years made me very aware of this inherent fragility we all have, but later on, I learned how to harness and channel all my mental horsepower to accomplish things I never thought possible for myself. And I did it by building what I now refer to as my Mental Lab.

Construction began after my last trip to Buffalo. That's when I finally stopped complaining long enough to realize the training ground that I needed was all around me. My messed-up life was the raw material I was looking for, and if I paid close attention to my impulses, insecurities, and actions, dropped the shame, and remained willing to dissect my self-doubt, anxiety, and fear, I would find the strength and motivation to transform my life.

Soon enough, I found myself hitting the books hard to prepare for the ASVAB test and spending six to eight hours in the gym or on the trails every day to qualify for Navy SEAL training. And it didn't take long to realize that, like life itself, difficult workouts and long study sessions tended to spotlight all my weak points. My desire to continue to eat crappy food, my natural impulse to cut corners in almost everything I did, my general lack of drive, and my flagging attention during those marathon ASVAB study sessions revealed my willingness to settle for mediocrity. But what came up for me most often was my failure in Pararescue training. It was my constant companion during those weeks. It shadowed me wherever I went.

I'd arrived at Air Force boot camp in the best shape of my life, and by the time Pararescue training began eight weeks later, I was in peak physical condition. I'd read the warning order front to back and prepared for each and every timed physical evolution, assuming my strength and speed would be enough. But I lacked the mental strength to see it through, and after a terrifying pool evolution, my fear of the water held me hostage until I quit. The more I dissected that situation, the more I realized how much I needed this new Mental Lab.

Being that I was almost three hundred pounds and had to lose more than one hundred in less than three months, I knew it wasn't possible to report to Naval Special Warfare Command in Coronado in the best physical shape of my life. But that wasn't necessary. My root problems were not and never had been physical. They were all mental.

In my Lab, each physical workout became a test of my mental fortitude. I stopped caring about how my body looked. You don't need six-pack abs when your mind is steel-plated. From that point on, each run, every hour on the pull-up bar, and all my late-night study sessions became experiments conducted to see how long my mind would hold out when I continued to apply more and more pressure. I was creating a man who was mentally prepared to do anything it took to become a SEAL. Even if it meant experiencing three Hell Weeks and running on broken legs.

Those same experiments continued for the next twenty years, and through all my countless trials, tumbles, and failures,

I cultivated an alter-ego—a savage who refused to quit under almost any circumstance. Someone capable of overcoming any and all obstacles. I felt compelled to share what I learned in the lab because I knew it could help people, and what started as a slow reveal of my inner drive on social media swelled to a deep confession in *Can't Hurt Me*. Anybody who tuned in or turned the page knew exactly where I came from and what drives me. But one thing I never shared was that there were two sides to my psyche and soul.

If you don't feel like you're good enough, if your life lacks meaning and time feels like it's slipping through your fingers, there is only one option. Recreate yourself in your own Mental Lab. Somewhere you can be alone with your thoughts and wrestle with the substance of what and who you want to be in your one short life on earth. If it feels right, create an alter ego to access some of that dark matter in your own mind. That's what I did. In my mind, David Goggins wasn't the savage who accomplished all the hard things. It was Goggins who did that.

David was the kid born with one eye closed and raised scared and shackled. There is nothing inherently special about me. I just stopped focusing on what was holding me back and learned to use rejection, pain, and failure as tools to harness every available bit of dark matter in my mind—all my unused strength, passion, and desire. It was rarely fun. I suffered way more than I smiled, but it helped me create my alter ego. Goggins was powered by the dark side of my soul that refused to be denied, and he had one goal: to become the hardest person to ever live!

We all have a Mental Lab at our disposal, but most people don't even know that they have access to a place where they can transform themselves. Therefore, they remain locked out. By the time they hit mid-life, the doors are wrapped with a rusty chain and deadbolted. The equipment inside is dusty and broken. Weeds are sprouting from the foundation and the roof.

For two decades, the doors to my Lab were locked too—because I'd locked myself inside! But after my heart scare, I realized that, without even knowing it, at some point, I'd sleepwalked out of my Mental Lab, and the doors had shut and locked behind me.

Then, on February 6, I received an email that twisted the knife. It came from Bob Babbitt, the man who introduced me to Greg Welch, one of the greatest triathletes ever, at the Ironman World Championship in 2008. Welch had undergone thirteen heart surgeries starting in his mid-thirties, which forced him into an early retirement. In my panicked state, I was sure this was some kind of bad omen, but Babbitt wrote to me with a simple question. He wanted to know if I'd consider running the Leadville Trail 100 later that summer to raise money for his charity, the Challenged Athletes Foundation (CAF).

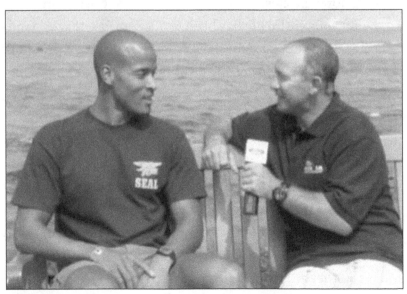

Being interviewed by the great Greg Welch at Kona Ironman 2008

Since 1994, the CAF has raised $134 million and funded thirty-five thousand athletes with physical challenges to get the coaching and support they need. It is a worthy cause to say the least, but it had been five years since my last 100-miler, when I DNF'd (did not finish) at Badwater, so I didn't reply right away. Instead, I stepped to the bathroom mirror and stared myself down. It wasn't Goggins staring back. It was David, and he was timid as hell.

I wondered if I would even be able to physically complete the race, let alone compete at the high level I had in so many ultra races during my prime. Those thoughts were painful because they told me that, although more than a month had passed since my trip to the ER, I was still a shell of my former self and felt fragile. I hadn't been cleared to train hard because the doctors still didn't know what was wrong with me, and as they put my heart through test after test, I remained low on motivation. After decades of hard charging, I was stuck in neutral, nowhere close to the mental beast I'd once been.

When your entire life has been riddled with setbacks, land-mines, and trap doors, some days, it's nearly impossible to find the motivation to keep getting after it. It's just too exhausting, and in that moment, I had no idea how much I had left in the tank. I searched my own eyes for an answer, a commitment, the last glowing embers of confidence from what used to be a raging inner fire.

If Badwater is the best-known ultra race on earth, the Leadville Trail 100 Run is a close second. The race begins and ends outside the old Rocky Mountain mining town of Leadville, Colorado, which is set at just over ten thousand feet above sea level and is rougher around the edges than the flashy ski resort and hippie towns nearby. The course is an out-and-back grind, with several major climbs combining for a total of over fifteen thousand vertical feet of elevation gain. I'd run Leadville once before, and I knew that fewer than half of all entrants are able to finish the race under the thirty-hour time limit. And those were runners without unidentified heart problems and sickle cell trait (which makes carriers more prone to altitude sickness). And when you live at sea level, training for a race at altitude is that much more difficult. Plus, with my speaking calendar packed to the limit, I knew I had months of travel and nothing but garbage training ahead of me. I'd be forced to run in strange cities down avenues with tons of stoplights and packed sidewalks or in residential areas I barely knew on roads peppered with four-way stops. For Leadville, ideal training isn't just optimal, it is required if you expect to pull off an acceptable personal performance.

Oh, I had plenty of convenient excuses to tap out. My hesitation was telling. My internal dialogue was trying to talk me out of a race I hadn't even fully considered. This is what the average mind does. The reasons to say no to something that we know will require our maximum dedication and promises no guarantee of success will bubble up two at a time until we give up before we even get started. That's when I knew I had already gone soft.

Sometimes, the biggest decisions in your life—the ones that will set your trajectory for weeks, months, years, or even decades to come—sneak up on you. I had so many valid reasons to turn Babbitt down flat, but I couldn't. Mostly because I could barely look at myself in the mirror and could not stand my weak tone.

Sure, I was busy, but I could make time to train. During my peak years in ultra racing, I had an event almost every weekend and still worked full-time. Back then, I had bolted the doors of my Mental Lab and lived there day and night. I signed up for 100-mile runs like they were forty-five-minute spin or HIIT classes. I put a range of obstacles in front of me just to gain the experience. As far as my health went, my heart hadn't given me any issues at all for ten years straight. I could use my Christmas trip to the ER as a crutch if I wanted to, but that's exactly what it was, and the fact that I was still leaning on that crutch told me there was something subversive at work in my psyche and soul.

"Is this what you've turned into?" I asked as I mad-dogged the man in the mirror. This wasn't the filthy, tarnished mirror of my youth. This one gleamed like crystal. "Some guy that wakes up to bacon and eggs, watches sports, delivers keynote presentations, and poses for pictures? You're not a savage. Not anymore. So, what are you?"

Professional fighters don't train for their biggest bouts at home. They head into the mountains or the woods, somewhere they can focus in relative isolation and without all the luxury. They don't bring their families. They bring their trainers, and every move they make is about rediscovering their primal nature and that hunger that made them hard and turned them into champions.

Back in my military days, I was a fighter who never broke camp. I stayed primal. What made me hard were the horrible tasks I stepped to and knocked off one at a time without hesitation. My daily goal was to wake up before anyone else. Sometimes, that meant 0500, sometimes 0400, and occasionally, I woke up at 0300 because I needed the first footprints in the sand or on the trail to be my own. If for some strange reason they weren't, I made sure that while they were sleeping at night, I was back out there grinding for two or three more hours. I was the unconditional competitor, a full-time savage. Then, things got comfortable, and I slipped into a new frame of mind.

All the effort I'd put into conquering my negative mind had changed me. My demons and insecurities, which had been my primary energy sources for two decades, no longer owned the same real estate in my brain. I had managed to finally put each of them in their rightful place, and in that vacuum, a new sense of self emerged. To write my book, I'd developed the mindset of an artist, and the book's great success was the one minefield I hadn't anticipated. While money doesn't always make you happy, it sure can make you feel satisfied. And satisfaction is a hop-step from complacency.

Oh, I looked the part. I was ripped, and if you tried to run with me, you'd come away thinking that I still had it. But even though I worked out twice a day, I was a part-time savage at best, a glorified Weekend Warrior. Weekend Warriors do hard things when they fit into their busy schedules. They do them to check a box and only when they want to. Then, they dial it back after a couple of long, hard days. When you are a full-time savage, it's a lifestyle. There is no "want to." There is only "must do." If I were still a true savage, still striving to be the hardest person to ever live, Babbitt's email wouldn't have inspired some soft, should-I-or-shouldn't-I inner debate. It would have lit a fuse.

While growth is important, you cannot lose the core of who you are. Your core is your stability. It's what dictates how you move through the world. Physically, when your core muscles are weak, you are literally a pushover. Psychologically, when your core values come into question, it's easy to lose yourself, and I could not afford to lose touch with the hard work it took to build this new life. But my Cookie Jar was stuffed with moldy cookies—stale victories from a different time that I couldn't relate to anymore. My Cookie Jar had always been an energy source, stocked with accomplishments that I could use to remind myself what I had overcome and was capable of. I knew I had to toss them all out and start fresh, but something inside me was still reluctant to reenter the crucible.

Mental toughness and resilience fade if they aren't used consistently. I say it all the time: you are either getting better, or you're getting worse. You're not staying the same. And I'd failed to heed my own words. I wasn't training to gain any longer. I had become a maintenance man, and while it's certainly possible to maintain muscle tone and a certain level of cardiovascular fitness, you cannot maintain the savage mind.

If you stop grabbing iron with your bare hands, they will lose their calluses. Your mind works the same way. You have to fight to keep that mindset of getting up every day to get after it because it wants to go away. Surgery, sickness, busy work schedules, and family commitments are all great excuses to take a rest today, which makes it that much easier to rest again tomorrow, and that's a slippery slope! The way I live and the things I do have always been about the mind. Long before the body goes soft, the mind will have softened. Fortunately, I wasn't that far gone, but my mind had softened a bit because I hadn't been challenged to the edge of my capabilities in years.

As much as I wanted to turn Babbitt down flat, I couldn't get Leadville out of my mind for days, and those days turned into weeks. The man's casual proposition had become my haunting, and the more I thought about my questionable heart, other lingering health issues, and my busy schedule, the less any of those variables seemed to matter. I had dealt with worse training, less sleep, and more travel in the military than I faced now. When I trained for Badwater the first time, my feet and ankles were so destroyed I couldn't even run for the first four weeks of training. I had to work out on the elliptical or with a rowing machine, and I never even considered letting injuries stop me. As winter turned to spring, I knew it was time to find my primal nature again, but I still didn't commit to Leadville.

For eight weeks, I lived in self-imposed purgatory. Depending on the minute, hour, or day, I told myself I was in and then enumerated all the valid reasons why it was best not to enter the race. Then, in April, after my cardiologist cleared me to train harder, I dipped my toe into the Leadville waters like the part-time savage I'd become. I didn't commit to Bob, but I did bump up my training…to a point. Instead of putting together a series of 100-mile weeks, I was content to clock in with fifties, but on those runs, my focus was way off. I hardly remembered anything I felt or saw out on the road.

This was unusual because unlike most people, I can't check out mentally when I run, and I don't use those miles to think about my to-do list. I have to stay locked in because I'm not a naturally gifted runner. The reason I can run at a relatively quick clip for a long time is due to my training volume but also because when I run, I focus on my stride, remain conscious of where and how my feet strike the ground and on my head and shoulder position. I visualize myself running with a tray of full water glasses on my head. I don't want any sway or bounce at all. I remain still yet relaxed and let my core and legs carry me forward.

Obviously, that amount of focus is tough to maintain for hours at a time. When I'm running well, I catalog every wrinkle in my form, each faulty foot strike. I can recall exactly where and when they happened and review them all in my mind's eye afterward. Because I don't run to burn calories or maintain cardiovascular fitness. To me, it's about achieving mental and physical greatness. The fact that I'd lost touch with that told me that I'd become just another runner, and I'd never been satisfied being just another anything.

If I wanted to crush Leadville and find myself again, I needed to demand more from myself on a daily basis. I had to sharpen my focus. I told Kish that I didn't want her to book any more speaking engagements. I have never been about the business aspect anyway, and while I appreciated all the respect and support from the people and organizations I engaged with, I knew it was having a corrosive effect on my mindset.

The ego is an amazing force. The more I heard about my own success, the more tempting it became to coast, as if I'd finally arrived. Even though I know that the journey never ends and that there is always more work to do, when life stops kicking you in the teeth and serves you a big bowl of praise pudding instead, it's easy to feel that you are the man. Especially if that level of respect was hard-earned. But praise—whether it comes from your supervisors, your family, or anyone else—has a downside. It can soothe the inner savage and keep you from feeling the need to grind.

My ego check had to include a moratorium on all things soft. I needed to break back into the Mental Lab and find the savage I used to be. I stopped taking most calls and texts. I tuned out and turned within. Which is another way of saying I put together a grueling ten-week, 1,200-mile training plan. Most people will tell you that 100-mile weeks are overkill because running that much for almost three months straight won't allow your body to recover properly. While ten miles a day had always been my sweet spot, I now had to tell my mind and body that I was no longer playing around. I needed that triple-digit mileage. I needed to land in Leadville knowing that I put the proper training in.

On June 4, I emailed Babbitt and told him that if there

was still space, I was willing to "race across the sky" for CAF. Part-time savage that I was, I emailed him three days after his deadline. Proof that Goggins was still MIA, and David was the one making all the moves. But Babbitt managed to get me in, and a week later, Kish and I landed in Avalon, New Jersey, for several weeks of training.

Avalon is on a pancake-flat, seven-mile-long island dotted with sprawling modern homes where Kish's family spends their summers on the sand. It's a pretty place filled with smiling families enjoying their summer vacations. The water is warm, the white-sand beaches are packed, and groups tend to gather on the bay to watch sunset each evening, soft serve ice cream cones in hand. Or so I'm told. I wouldn't know. I spent my time out on the road.

I ran fifteen to twenty-five miles every day in the muggy East Coast summer heat. Training at altitude wasn't an option, so peak heat and humidity at sea level would have to do. Most days, I crisscrossed the island multiple times to get my miles in. I never checked the weather before I left the house, and at first, I carried a single water bottle with me but quickly learned that wasn't nearly enough. After an hour, that bottle would be empty, and I had to finish the run dry.

I experimented with my hydration the best I could. I tried carrying two bottles. I staged the course by dropping bottles in the bushes, but by Independence Day, when the heat cranked up above ninety degrees and the humidity index rose above 85 percent, those bottles were heating up so much they were worthless. I went back to carrying just the one bottle. After I drained it, my hydration plan was the same one I used on long runs in the tropics back in my military days. Whenever I got thirsty, I licked my damn lips.

Humidity and hydration weren't my only problems in Avalon. There were pests. I ran through clouds of ravenous mosquitoes, and down by the water, I dealt with the island's notorious greenheads—biting flies that wouldn't leave me alone. Oh, and don't let me forget the attack birds. It was just my luck that red-winged blackbirds nest in Avalon every summer, usually on the quiet inland roads I preferred. Whenever I came within a quarter mile of any nest, a bird flew at me and tried to bury its talons into my scalp. They circled, squawked, and dove until I was out of their territory. Of course, there were miles of nests and dozens of angry birds. After a few days, I learned to take off my shirt well ahead of time so I could swing it at those feathered beasts to keep the dive bombers at bay. Yessir, we were a sight to behold.

The weeks progressed, and the conditions deteriorated. And that's when I began to enjoy myself. Some days, I left the house without breakfast and after barely eating dinner the night before. I wanted to run my daily twenty bonked because I knew a moment like that was bound to come in the Rocky Mountains. I needed to train the body to churn out miles even after the fuel tank was drained and send a message to myself that I was capable of finding energy where there was none.

One afternoon, I hit a wall at mile fifteen. My pace plummeted from seven minutes per mile to the mid-nines. I was out of water, of course. But as miserable as it was, I found myself enjoying being dizzy, dehydrated, and calorie-starved. I relished the suffering because it let me know that I still had it in me to push myself that hard, and I scorched the final mile in seven minutes flat.

One of the hottest days of the year was in mid-July, when the mercury climbed above one hundred degrees and the humidity was over 80 percent. The heat index was off the charts, and the air quality was horrible too. The county issued a warning advising residents to remain indoors. In Gogglish, that meant it was the perfect day for a twenty-two-mile run.

Avalon is always bumping during the month of July, when the bike lane is heavily trafficked and the pancake houses and bakeries have long lines of eager customers. That day, the streets were silent. For ten miles, I didn't see anybody at all. In the eleventh mile, a car crept past me ever so slowly, and I could tell the driver recognized me. Sure enough, he flipped a U-turn and came rolling right up beside me.

"David Goggins! Man, I knew that was you!" I glanced over at him. He looked reasonably fit and athletic. He was also baffled, and maybe even a little concerned, as he watched me pound the pavement. "Dude, why are you even out here on a day like this?" I shrugged and shook my head.

"Because you're not."

I didn't think much of my flippant comment at first. But as I ran ahead, I savored it. I'd picked the worst day of the summer for my longest run of the week. Why? Because nobody else would even consider doing something like that, and that gave me a chance to prove myself to be uncommon amongst the uncommon once again. I wasn't exactly the savage from SEAL training, but I was closer than I'd been in years.

I ran on in a state of mind that I hadn't experienced since Strolling Jim, a Tennessee road race I won in 2016. I'd attacked that course with calm focus and ran those 41.2 miles like it was a marathon, at a 7:07 per mile pace. I tracked down the race leader with eight miles to go, then held on to finish in under five hours and win by three minutes. In the brutal heat of Avalon, I discovered that same state of mind and body and realized that the man I thought I'd buried with too much comfort and success was still inside me, waiting to be unleashed.

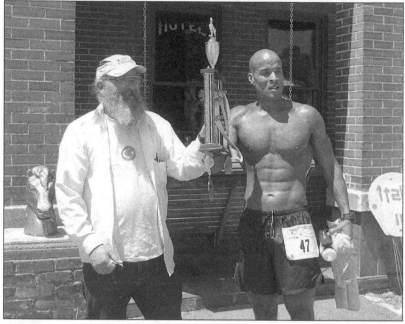

On the comeback at Strolling Jim...or so I thought

The world needs doctors, lawyers, and teachers, but we also need savages to prove that we are all capable of so much more. After ten weeks of hard-charging and eight weeks of heat training, I was well on my way to rediscovering something I thought I'd lost.

EVOLUTION NO. 3

Many dreams die while suffering. Think about it. We conjure our biggest dreams, our most audacious goals, when we feel safe and warm. Even if you're struggling financially, emotionally, spiritually, or physically, your grand plan to defy the odds probably came to you in a moment of comfort, when you had time to evaluate where you are and how you got there. There is no space for big-picture thinking when you're in the heat of battle. When all is calm, even temporarily, damn near anything can feel possible. So that's when you dream it up and map it all out.

Then you begin and unforeseen challenges knock you back. Whenever you're engaged in an intense struggle, the result of which will have a major impact on your life going forward, you will be challenged to your utmost—and these moments of truth within a larger quest can demand so much from you that you are bound to feel overmatched at times. When that happens, many people panic because they come to believe that they are imposters and their dream was actually a fantasy. In a blink, they go from being driven and focused to becoming convinced that they had no business even trying. So they quit. Right then. Right there. While teetering on the edge, they fail to grasp that there is something they can do to jam that quitter's spiral carrying them right down the drain.

They can make the One-Second Decision to think instead of react.

During my second Hell Week, when I was in Class 231, I was driven. Bill Brown and I were the leaders of Boat Crew Two, and we had our own competition going to see who would be the baddest man in the whole class. But there was another guy in the mix who had captured my attention—let's call him Mora. He was about our size, strong and fit, and whenever things got hard on the beach or the Grinder, he gravitated toward me. He was not in our boat crew yet wanted to feed off of my energy because Bill Brown and I were performing at such a high level, we made hell look and feel not only manageable but easy.

On day two of Hell Week, Mora found me in the chow hall with a lost look on his face and fear in his eyes. I was busy filling my wet and sandy pockets with packets of peanut butter because I needed fuel to withstand the punishment I knew was coming. Even after consuming as many calories as I could, in two hours, I'd be hungry again and would eat almost anything, even peanut butter gritty with sand and laced with pocket lint. Mora stared at me as if I were a creature from a different time, and I was. I'd become wholly uncivilized after two days of surf torture and boat runs without a wink of sleep. I was now a caveman. Mora, on the other hand, looked like a traumatized modern man, and that was a clue that something was off.

"Hey, Goggins," he whispered as his eyes darted around the room. "I don't wanna be here anymore." The pressure cooker of Hell Week had temporarily unhinged him from his dream and his rational mind, and he looked like he was searching for an emergency exit. He was panic in human form, and I knew that because it was exactly how I felt when the first wave hit me in the very first hour of that same Hell Week.

The Pacific Ocean was as cold as ever when that massive, six-foot wall of water picked me up, flipped me three times, and pounded me into the wet sand. It was as if the ocean itself was saying, "Get the hell out of here!" And I listened because my lungs were still burning from the bout of pneumonia that got me rolled into this class from Class 230 just two months earlier, and because water was my kryptonite.

There were 130 hours of Hell Week to come, and I knew that a good chunk of them would be spent in the cold ocean. That cocktail of suck hijacked my brain to send out signals far more troubling than ambivalence. I wasn't wondering if I had what it took or if I was prepared for the moment. The voice in my head was saying, *I don't really want to be a Navy SEAL.*

For more than a year, my quest to become a SEAL had been all-consuming. I'd never wanted anything as badly or committed so completely to the process, but when you are locked into a sufferfest, there are times when the conditions will become intolerable, and a self-sabotaging impulse rooted in shock and fear will feel like clarity. I was a half-step from voluntarily pulling the plug on a dream that had the power to change the course of my entire life.

I glanced over at Bill Brown, resigned to the fact that he would soon stand alone as the baddest man in Class 231. Then, from the knee-deep, swirling shallows, I scanned the horizon, where a destroyer was heading out to sea. The instructors had warned us that if we didn't make it through training, we'd be assigned to a ship like that, where we'd be stuck chipping paint for six months at a time. They made it sound like the most miserable deployment on earth, but to me, in that instant, it sounded like heaven.

Most SEAL instructors love quitters. When you tell them that you're too cold and you want out, they are more than happy to take you by the hand and lead you to the warmest shower of your life because, in their minds, it proves that they are better than you. Once you step into that shower, you get so warm within a minute that you forget what being cold even felt like, and then, you realize that your warmth just cost you a piece of your soul, if not the whole thing, which can lead to a lifetime of regret.

Time was of the essence! I could not crawl back onto the beach and take ten minutes to get my mind right. I was in the eye of a psychological storm, and all around me, the water was still frothing and growling. Part of the problem was that the cold water had stolen the breath from my lungs. I was gasping and panic-breathing. In order to think clearly, I needed oxygen. I took a deep breath and then another, and in that time, my possible future played out in my head.

I watched myself stagger back to the beach and lay my helmet down. Within days, I was flushed right out of the military and sent back to Indiana, where I struggled through a series of low-level, low-impact jobs, which were the only ones I was qualified for: minimum-wage security guard, lifeguard at a local pool, and exterminator. That was true clarity. All my aspirations would be vaporized if I left surf torture behind because I was a reservist, and if I snapped and quit, the Navy wouldn't even want me on one of their ships.

I could not afford to lose control. SEAL training—and that cold ocean—were exactly where I belonged, so I needed to calm down and meet the challenge head-on. I took another breath as the next big wave swelled. It smashed me, but I managed to scramble toward the group and lock arms with my teammates. I was done showing weakness. I was finished with fear. I would stay in that water as long as it took!

When we got called back onto the sand ten minutes later, the men in my boat crew were shivering and stiff. They were so cold they didn't even want the edges of their soaked T-shirts to graze their skin. We needed to warm up fast, and the only way to do that during Hell Week is to go hard. I nodded to Bill, grabbed the front of the boat, and shouted out orders. As a unit, Boat Crew Two started putting out like Hell Week was our natural habitat.

Often, it's the shock that launches the spin-out. For me, it was the snap of the cold water that triggered my fight-or-flight response, which comes with an adrenaline rush that spikes the heart and respiratory rates and puts your insecurities on blast. Your body and mind react that way because they want to protect you by telling you to remove yourself from the suffering. Fight or flight is exactly what Mora was experiencing in the chow hall. His fear and panic owned him.

When I was teetering on the brink, I was able to physically calm myself down with a few deep breaths, and that helped me see through the adrenaline rush. My heart rate was still elevated, and panic continued to creep in, but I'd regained enough of my composure to make a conscious One-Second Decision to stay in the fight. That took mental fortitude because the water hadn't suddenly warmed up. I was still cold and miserable and staring at 130 hours of Hell. But I was able to see that the life

I desired was on the other side of surf torture. I did not cave into emotion and quit. When people do that, they aren't even making an actual decision to quit. It's a default reaction due to stress.

I get that it's difficult not to give in to all that emotion, acute pain, and discomfort. All you really want at that point is for it to end. You envision your bed at home and how sweet it feels to lie down with your wife or husband or partner. You know your mom will greet you with a forgiving hug and that your family will understand because they love you no matter what. You know for a fact that they will console and take care of you, and when you're hurting bad or scared to death, all of that feels way too good to pass up.

But you must remember that those images of home aren't actually rooted in love. They are a product of your fear, disguised as love. Mora and I shared the same big dream. We'd both had our worlds rocked. I recovered by dominating Hell Week in a fashion that nobody had seen before. Mora's mind had already unraveled by the time I saw him in the chow hall. He wasn't thinking consciously at all. His emotions were controlling him instead of the other way around. I couldn't help him because by then, he'd already lost the battle. I don't know when he officially quit. In Hell Week, you get so wrapped up in your crew, so engulfed in helping one another get to the other side that, after several hours, you might look up and find half the class has bailed out. All I know is that, at some point, he rang the bell and lived to regret it.

Everything in life comes down to how we handle those crucial seconds. When psychological, physical, or emotional pressure redlines, your adrenal glands go haywire, and you are no longer in control. What separates a true savage from everybody else is the ability to regain control of their mind in that split second, despite the fact that all looks lost!

That's what people miss. Our lives aren't built on hours, days, weeks, months, or years. Hell Week is 130 hours, but it's not the hours that kill you. And it's not the pain, the exhaustion, or the cold. It is the 468,000 seconds that you must win. It only takes one of those seconds—when it all becomes too much and you just can't take it anymore—to bring you down. I had to remain vigilant and manage my mind for every single one of those seconds to make it.

Life, like Hell Week, is built on seconds that you must win, repeatedly. I'm not saying you have to be hyperaware every second of your life, but if you are pursuing something that demands all you've got and means the world to you, that is often what it takes.

When you are trying to lose weight or quit drinking or using drugs, your moment of weakness can be counted in seconds, and you'll need to be ready to win those seconds. You could be the medical student who has dreamed of being a doctor their entire life, only to fail a crucial class early on. Overwhelmed with panic, you may be tempted to march straight to the admissions office and withdraw. Maybe you are an aspiring lawyer with a job at a prestigious firm in your back pocket yet failed the bar exam again, and in the heat of that moment, you abandon your career before it begins. All because you become convinced that you cannot walk back into that office after another humiliation or study for that test again and put yourself right back on the chopping block.

While school and professional exams are held in controlled environments, an F can spike the heart rate and trigger self-doubt as quickly as a six-foot wall of cold water. Sometimes, that grade looms so large, especially in a young mind, that it's easy to feel like all eyes are on you and your failure and that you've fallen so far behind that you'll never catch up.

Moments of doubt are unavoidable when we take on any strenuous task. I've used the One-Second Decision to regain my composure and win hundreds of small battles during ultra races, on the pull-up bar, and in stressful work situations. And the first step is to mentally take a knee.

The best person in any combat scenario is the one who is composed enough to take a knee when the bullets are flying at them. They know they need to evaluate the situation and the landscape to find a way forward and that it's impossible to make a conscious decision if they or their team is running around like fire ants. Taking a knee in battle is not as easy as it sounds, but it's the only way to give yourself time to breathe through the panic and rein in your spinning mind so you are able to operate. The battle hasn't stopped. Gunfire is still lighting up the night, and you don't have any time to waste. In that one second, you must take a breath and decide to bring the fight.

When you are in the grip of life and in danger of losing control, just think, *It's time to take a knee.* Get a couple of breaths and flash to your future. If you fold, what will happen next? What's your plan B? This is not some deep contemplation. There is no time to order a pizza and hash it out with your people. This must happen in seconds!

It helps to prepare with productive self-talk before you drop into that sufferfest on your schedule. Remind yourself that nobody is great at every single aspect of any job, at least not right away, and no runner skates through a hard race unchallenged. No matter how bleak it looks or feels, you must stay rooted to your baseline.

If you're in med school, your baseline is to graduate and become a doctor. In Coronado, my baseline was becoming a Navy SEAL. Many men buckled under the log during Hell Week, but log PT was easy for me. I had to remember that every time we were ordered back into my own personal torture chamber, the Pacific Ocean.

It helps to remind yourself of what you're good at and where you excel so when you have to engage in something that is hard for you, it doesn't become overwhelming. Tell yourself, *I'm good here. I'm great there. This sucks, but it will be over in twenty minutes.* Maybe it's twenty miles or twenty days or twenty weeks, but it doesn't matter. Every experience on earth is finite. It will end someday, and that makes it doable, but the outcome hinges on those crucial seconds you must win!

There are consequences to this stuff. Quitting on a dream stays with you. It can color how you see yourself and the decisions you make going forward. Several men have taken their own lives after quitting SEAL training. Others marry the first person who comes around because they are so desperate for validation. Of course, the reverse is also true. If you can withstand the suffering, take a knee, and make a conscious One-Second Decision in a critical juncture, you will learn perseverance and gain strength by winning the moment. You will know what it takes and how it feels to overcome all that loud doubt, and that will stay with you too. It will become a powerful skill you can use again and again to find success, no matter what scenario you're in or where life takes you.

It's not always the wrong move to quit. Even in battle, sometimes we must retreat. You might not be ready for whatever it is you've taken on. Perhaps your preparation wasn't as thorough as you'd thought. Maybe other priorities in life need your attention. It happens, but make sure that it is a conscious decision you're making, not a reaction. Never quit when your pain and insecurity are at their peak. If you must retreat, quit when it's easy, not when it's hard. Control your thought process and get through the most difficult test first. That way, if you do bow out, you'll know it wasn't a reaction based on panic. Instead, you've made a conscious decision based on reason and had time to devise your plan B.

Mora quit on impulse. Usually when you do that, you don't get another chance. Many great opportunities in life only come around once, but sometimes, opportunity does knock twice. Fifteen months after that morning in the chow hall, we crossed paths in Coronado again. It was my graduation day, and he was in our Hooyah class, the incoming trainees wearing the white shirts that signified Day One, Week One. Of all the two hundred and some newbies, he was the only man there who wasn't smiling. He alone knew too much. After the ceremony, he approached, extended his hand, and congratulated me.

"Remember," I said, "many dreams die while suffering, bro." He nodded once, then faded into the crowd. A month later, I heard he made it through Hell Week. Five months after that, he graduated and became a Navy SEAL.

I thought about Mora as I gazed into my pristine, polished mirror twenty-two years later while considering Babbitt's invitation to Leadville. I'd been living large for longer than I cared to admit. In this new life of mine, the water was never cold and the One-Second Decision was in danger of becoming a perishable skill. I didn't think I needed it anymore. I had access to all the finer things. In my house, it was always seventy-two degrees. And that feels good, especially when you believe you've earned it.

Why put myself through a ten-week training camp or a 100-mile run in Colorado's thin air? I knew how horrible that experience is and what it takes, but I also knew that this right here was one of the most important One-Second Decisions in my life. This wasn't a fight-or-flight moment. I wasn't overwhelmed by the fear of death. I wasn't on the brink of failure or humiliation, and my heart rate was beating slow and steady. This was a mature version of the unconscious impulse to quit. The one you don't see coming until it greets you at the gate when you think you've finally arrived.

See, I don't have any respect for people who live this luxe life 24/7. If I said no to Babbitt, I wouldn't be quitting on him. I would be quitting on myself. I would be making a fear-based choice to no longer be the very person who I became so proud of. It's all well and good to have success and reach a certain level, but I really don't care what you did yesterday. Maybe you finished Ultraman or graduated from Harvard. I do not care. Respect is earned every day by waking up early, challenging yourself with new dreams or digging up old nightmares, and embracing the suck like you have nothing and have never done a damn thing in your life.

> There are 86,400 seconds in a day. Losing just one of those seconds can change the outcome of your day and, potentially, your life. #OneSecondDecision #NeverFinished

CHAPTER FOUR

A SAVAGE REBORN

Two weeks before the race, Kish and I flew into Aspen to acclimatize, but after a week of two-a-days, including long trail runs in the morning and daily speed hikes up Ajax Mountain each afternoon, my body was in shutdown mode. I wasn't sleeping well, and my lungs felt torched. Even walking up the stairs left me winded. My legs were knotted up so tight that I had no turnover at all. Kish shadowed me on every run and noticed that my pace was declining each day. In our hotel room after yet another disappointing training session, she sensed my frustration.

"You don't need to do this to yourself, David," she said. "You've run this race before. If you never enter another race in your life, you will still have done more than most people can even dream of doing."

I sat on the edge of the bed and turned to her. I could see the concern in her eyes. She still hadn't gotten over my latest heart scare, and it was painful for her to watch the thin air jack me up. But all I could think about was the last time I'd signed up for a 100-miler.

It was Badwater 135 in July 2016. I'd been stretching two hours a day for a few years by then, and as my muscles grew more pliable, I became convinced I was unlocking more mental and physical potential. I'd won Strolling Jim in Tennessee in early May and was confident when I drove up to Death Valley a few weeks before Badwater to get a training run in. But seven miles into that run, the heat became so intense that my pulse skyrocketed, and then the craziest thing happened. I stopped.

I was the guy who'd savored scorching temperatures. I'm not beating any world-class runner based on speed alone, but if it's a hot sufferfest, I have a chance. That's how I'd always thought, yet there had been a sudden glitch in my operating system, and that mentality was "file not found." When race day came around, I was nowhere near Badwater Basin, the start line of the race.

"Do you want me to call the guys?" Kish asked. I'd lined up two friends to crew the race. They were hours away from boarding their flights. "Should I cancel their trips and tell them Leadville is off?"

Kish was right that given how I felt physically, one hundred unnecessary miles at altitude seemed like the very definition of a very bad idea. And now, she was telling me I was one phone call away from salvation, and I wouldn't even have to make it myself. However, while my body was most definitely jacked up, my mind was starting to harden up.

This was not 2016! So what if my legs weren't churning, Kish could hang with me on every run, or Ajax repeatedly kicked my butt? Altitude wasn't my problem. The only issue I could see was that I hadn't run a 100-mile race in five years, and I'd forgotten that feeling worn out before a race was status quo for me. I'd never tapered before any of my events back in the day, which meant I never once showed up to the start line with loose, rested legs. Whether I came in first, second, third, or last made no difference to me back then. I'd once walked one hundred miles to finish Badwater, and if I had to, I'd do it again in Leadville.

In other words, everything was in its rightful place. Even with my physical fitness faltering, my mind was gaining strength with every hour spent on the trails. I was starting to think like a savage again and banking knowledge that I had successfully climbed steep terrain at altitude, despite how I felt, so that I could lean on that experience to keep me feeling confident, even when I was uncomfortable, undernourished, sleep deprived, and dehydrated and on the steepest, hardest climbs of the Leadville course.

An unprepared mind prefers a proper taper and rested legs. It prays for a clear, sixty-degree race-day morning and a tailwind that flows in both directions. And maybe a little drizzle every third mile, but only for a few seconds, to cool off. Not enough to make the trail muddy or slick.

A prepared mind craves the worst conditions because it knows that pressure brings out its best and exposes almost everyone else. It doesn't care if your legs are working right, if the temperature is perfect, if there is one miserable hill or an entire mountain range waiting to crush you. When there are freezing river crossings, it doesn't concern itself with your wet feet. It doesn't pay any attention to distance, and it sure doesn't give a damn how long it takes to get there. The prepared mind is a magnificent thing, and mine was just about ready. My nutrition plan was dialed in, and my self-talk and visualization were on point. And you know what that guaranteed me?

Absolutely nothing!

So much had changed since my last race. These events used to be my time away from humanity. It was the place I went to enter an animal state of body and mind, and it was easy to disappear because not many people were into the sport. Back in the early 2000s, there were only about twenty or so 100-mile events in the entire calendar year, raced by a hard-core crew of runners hungry for some suffering. You could rock up on the day of the race and gain entry. Now, there are more than two hundred 100-mile races each year in the United States alone. Ultra running had gone mainstream during my absence, and the start line for Leadville was surreal. The field was packed with over eight hundred happy, chatty athletes taking selfies and streaming live.

The energy was palpable as we shook loose, preparing to tackle an out-and-back course, most of it on the Colorado Trail, which ranges between 9,200 feet and 12,600 feet in elevation. Most of us weren't trying to win. Typically, less than half the field completes the course within the designated thirty-hour time limit.

I'd learned long ago that no matter what type of event or challenge I engage in, the only competition that ever matters is me against me. A lot of people will take that as yet another invitation to coast. Please don't. Though I hadn't entered a 100-mile race in years, I planted a carrot—something to chase—in the back of my mind to keep my focus dialed in. Life is not pass/fail. It's about impact and effort. Carrots help me maximize both and almost always produce a better result. If I was going to do Leadville, I was going to do Leadville to the best of my ability. No matter how bad I felt physically, I didn't come all the way out here just to see if I could finish in thirty hours. My goal was to finish in under twenty-four.

It took a few miles to get warmed up, but I was pleasantly surprised with my pace and form. My race plan was the same as usual. I would speed-hike the ups and run the flats and downs. Most ultra runners use that strategy because running steep inclines burns your reserves, and you don't really make up that much time. During a long event like Leadville, it's better to spend your energy elsewhere.

I had scouted the course thoroughly in the days before the race, looking for any edge. Not only to become reacquainted with the terrain but also so Kish knew how to get to where she and the rest of the crew needed to be. We visited the sites set to become aid stations and mapped everything out, leaving nothing to chance. My preparation was on point, but when you're exhausted in the Rockies, no matter how well you've scouted a trail, it's easy to get tricked into thinking you've reached the top of the pass when you aren't even close.

The Leadville Trail 100 has a bunch of false summits. The most infamous one is on Hope Pass at 12,600 feet above sea level. The climb begins at around the forty-mile mark, and it's the last major pass before the turnaround at Winfield. By then, I'd found a rhythm, and my legs were still in decent shape despite having put in more miles that day than I had in three years. As the singletrack trail snaked steadily up toward the tree line, I speed-hiked by pressing my hands on my knees for leverage, while the vast majority of the other runners around me used trekking poles. I was an old-school ultra guy. To me, those poles looked like crutches. I was content going hands on knees all the way to the top. Nevertheless, poles were allowed, and they do make you faster. I could tell because I kept losing ground as the trail wound higher and higher.

After a few miles, the trail poked out above tree line and

leveled off in the tundra. It looked and felt like we'd reached the top, and I saw several runners get happy. Pleased enough to pick up their pace, but as soon as we rounded the next bend and saw how much there was still left to climb, their heads dropped, and their shoulders slumped, while I smiled to myself and kept grinding. Bent at the waist, my palms pressed onto my knees, driving more power into the balls of my feet as they struck the ground, which allowed me to chop the climb down to size, one step at a time.

People who've spent time on high country trails know the heartbreak of a false summit. When all you want is for the incline to stop kicking your butt, it tricks you into thinking you've made it, only to reveal that you aren't even close! But you don't have to be a trail rat to know that feeling. In life, there are plenty of false summits.

Maybe you think you've rocked an assignment at work or school, only to have your teacher or supervisor rip it to pieces or tell you to start over again. False summits can come in the gym when you're doing a hard circuit workout and think you've hit the last set, only to hear from your coach or trainer—or from a quick glance at your own notes—that you have to go back through the entire circuit one last time. We all take a punch like that every once in a while, but those who tend to crane their necks looking for the crest of the mountain as they beg for their suffering to end are the ones who get smashed the most by any false summit.

We have to learn to stop looking for a sign that the hard time will end. When the distance is unknown, it is even more critical that you stay locked in so the unknown factor doesn't steal your focus. The end will come when it comes, and anticipation will only distract you from completing the task in front of you to the best of your ability. Remember, the struggle is the whole journey. That's why you're out there. It's why you signed up for this race, or that class, or took the job. There is great beauty when you are involved in something that is so hard most people want it to end. When Hell Week ended, most of the guys who survived cheered, wept tears of joy, high-fived, or hugged one another. I got the Hell Week blues because I'd been immersed in the beauty of grinding through it and the personal growth that came with it.

We can make any obstacle as big or small as we like. It's all in the way we frame it. Going into Leadville, I expected one long, hard day. But how many inconsequential days had I lived by then? Why not spend one single day doing something I'll be proud of for the rest of my life? Like Elmo said to Louden Swain in his apartment before the wrestling match of his life in the movie *Vision Quest*, "It ain't the six minutes. It's what happens in that six minutes."

When you're climbing a mountain or involved in any other difficult task, the only way to free yourself from the struggle is to finish it. So why whine about it when it gets hard? Why hope it will end soon when you know it will end eventually? When you complain and your mind starts groping for the eject button, you are not bringing your best self to the task, which means you are actually prolonging the pain.

The hard chargers keep their heads down and hammer away. They have trained their minds to stay hard in those hard moments. They recognize the false summit for what it is and will always act as if they are nowhere near the top. Most people slow down and suffer on a steep trail, but slope and elevation are of no consequence to the hard charger. They keep their mind in attack mode until there are no more mountains to climb, and when they actually reach the top, they wish it had lasted a little bit longer.

After about four miles of climbing, I jogged through the dip between two peaks at Hope Pass and shook my head. *Over already?* I thought as I picked up the pace and hammered the descent toward the turnaround at mile fifty, where my crew was waiting.

I was just off my Leadville PR pace of twenty-two hours and fifteen minutes, which put me in the top forty in the entire field. Not that I knew that at the time. I didn't wear a fitness watch. I wore a ten-dollar special from Walmart that I bought the day before because I didn't want knowledge of my pace clouding my mindset. I was focused on one thing: the task at hand.

After a short rest to eat and hydrate, it was time to retrace my steps and climb up Hope Pass from the backside, this time with a pacer. My old friend T. J. had stuffed his pack with the extra food, water, and gear he thought I might need, and his legs were fresh. His presence pushed me up that ascent at a strong pace, and although it had been some time since I'd run trails consistently, I had become a good technical trail runner over the years. That muscle memory clicked back in, which enabled me to attack the descent and fly down the other side.

The final major climb in the race loomed at mile seventy-five. It's called Powerline, and that one has a few false summits too. T. J. had a pair of trekking poles with him, and he kept offering them to me. He had been annoyed watching people with poles pass us on the backside of Hope Pass while I was still hiking hands on knees. We caught most of them on the way down and on the flats, only to give up ground again on Powerline.

"Come on, man, just try the poles for a mile or two," he said. "See if you like 'em."

"Screw that," I snapped, as two more people passed us up. "In the old days, that was cheating." I was cooked by then. For the first time all day, the accumulated miles and my pace were starting to wear on me, and he could see it.

"I'm telling you, Goggins." I looked over as T. J. held them out like he knew he was presenting a weapon of last resort to a grumpy samurai still clinging to the old ways. I snatched them, irritated that I was abandoning the old ultra ethic. Then again, the sport had evolved, and this was an opportunity for me to evolve with it. As he promised, those poles took so much pressure off my legs they suddenly felt fresh, and I charged up that steep mountain.

I was moving better and faster than I had in several hours. I passed seasoned ultra runners like so many slalom flags. My confidence swelled and my senses heightened as I moved up in the field. I felt so powerful and in the flow that something shook loose in my memory and tumbled to the front of my mind. That's what makes events like Leadville so deep and poetic. A 100-mile grind at altitude will wring everything out of you, and as I flew up Powerline, I saw the scared kid who used to look for exits because he was blind to his own possibilities.

❊ ❊ ❊

My stuttering surfaced midway through third grade in my second year in Brazil, Indiana. By the time I was in fifth, I couldn't say three words without stammering. It was especially bad around grown-ups and strangers and at its absolute worst when public speaking was involved. I'll never forget the school play. Everyone knew I stuttered, but since participation was mandatory, my teacher mercifully assigned me a role with just one line. I practiced it at home a hundred times. Sometimes, I'd stumble. Usually, it came out smooth and wrinkle-free, but under those stage lights, I locked up.

The silence was intolerable. There were fifteen, twenty people in attendance at most, all of them were parents, and you couldn't ask for a more supportive audience. Everyone waited patiently, almost willing me to speak. A few of my classmates snickered, but most were rooting for me. My teacher watched with wide, sensitive eyes as my lower lip trembled. I knew it was hopeless, so I turned and left the stage without even trying.

I went to a small Catholic school. Everyone in my grade had known me for years, and I was relatively comfortable around them. Most had been there when my stuttering began midway through third grade, and they'd watched it mutate into a curse I couldn't escape when I was asked to read aloud in class. Sometimes, I had to read a couple of sentences, especially when we were learning the definitions of new words. Often, it would be a paragraph or two, which made it even worse because then not only was my stammering an issue, but the fact that I struggled to read was also on blast.

In those moments, time stopped, and I felt completely exposed. It didn't matter that my curse had been nourished by past trauma and the anxiety of being the only Black kid in a White school. In my mind, I was now the stupid Black kid who stuttered and nothing more. My failure felt heavier than it actually was, and my anxiety around public speaking only grew. It got to the point where whenever the teacher called on us to read aloud, one after another, I would count paragraphs ahead, and at the most strategic moment, ask for a bathroom break. Unless I faked a headache or nausea to get sent home for the rest of the day.

My entire existence in that school was built around avoiding exposure. It wasn't about studying or improving. It was about dodging bullets because all I could see was incoming fire, which limited my ability to learn and grow. I started cheating to keep up because my stuttering convinced me I couldn't hang in the classroom and that there was nothing for me in those schoolbooks.

My last thoughts before I fell asleep each night and my first upon waking were of my own insignificance, stupidity, and worthlessness. Due to my hard upbringing, I was more aware of how the world worked than most fifth graders, and I couldn't help but wonder how I was going to get through life if I couldn't get a word out. What became of people like that? The thought terrified me. My world was closing in because my stuttering ruled me. It was all I could see, hear, and feel. There was no available space for any positive thought to take root in my brain. So, I gravitated toward shortcuts and hunted emergency exits.

For many people, the haunting begins the minute they wake up. Maybe they are fat or disabled, feel ugly, or are failing and overwhelmed at school or work, and it consumes them. Their obsession with their own imperfections and faults suffocates self-respect and submarines progress, and from the time they get out of bed until they are able to crawl back in that night, the only thing on their agenda is avoiding exposure and surviving another day in hell. When that's how you feel about yourself, it's impossible to see possibilities or seize opportunities.

We all have the ability to be extraordinary, but most of us—and especially the haunted ones—tap out of the crucible and never experience what it's like to get to the other side of hell. My metamorphosis was a brutal process that unfolded over decades, but eventually, I became the polar opposite of the kid frozen in the hot stage lights and the gaze of his teacher who only wanted to teach him to read. I became a full-time savage who walked the distant, narrow path with cliffs rising on both sides, no aid stations or rest areas, and no turnouts or exits of any kind. Whatever popped up in front of me had to be dealt with head-on because the full-time savage sees everything in life as an opportunity to learn, adapt, and evolve. However, when Babbitt's message found me, at first, I looked for an exit. Then, I got my head back in the game and found a way.

Now, over seventy-five miles into one of the most difficult races on earth, I felt unnaturally strong, which is exactly why those images from my fifth-grade play continued to run on a loop in my mind's eye. Your strongest moments will often make you think of your weakest. I was pushing so hard my perspective ran deep, and I felt for that kid, knowing he allowed situations to dominate him for way too long. But I was proud of him too. For overcoming all of that. It is truly amazing what that little kid accomplished.

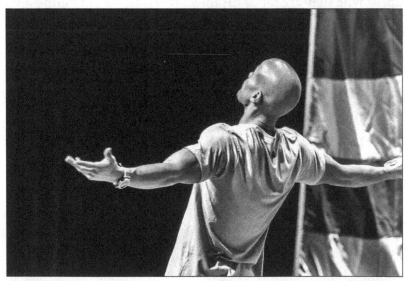

On stage speaking at The Patriot Tour, no longer afraid of stuttering (credit to Nature's Eye)

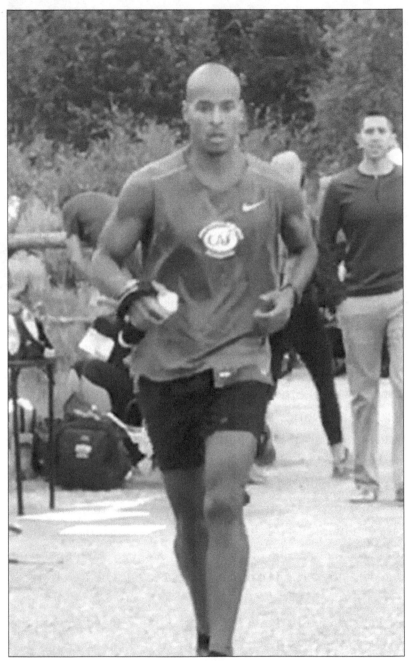

After twelve years, it feels good to be back at **Leadville.**

The descent from Powerline is on a fire road sprayed with so many rocks and boulders it's difficult to find sure footing, but I made good time. From then on, whenever the trail leveled off, I ran. When the incline cranked back up, I used poles and hiked faster than I ever had before.

Leadville was a purging of my soul. All the questions I had coming into the event about my inner drive and physical ability were answered. It was as if the high-altitude racecourse itself was a sculptor, and I was its marble masterpiece in progress: the image of a savage reborn. Every mile I ran, another chunk of rock fell away, and I came into the final aid station at mile eighty-seven thinking how crazy it was that a few days earlier, it looked like I might have to walk the whole thing. Now, with just thirteen miles to go, my legs still had a lot left.

During my time in the aid station, I absorbed the scene. Some runners staggered in. Others laughed and joked with their crews while they ate and rehydrated. All of us were almost through a barbaric rite of passage, but after it was all over, how many would use it as an opportunity to ask deeper questions of their body and mind and demand more of themselves? Leadville 2019 was populated with plenty of part-time savages. People who dial up their training for six or seven months, complete a race of a lifetime, and then sit back and do nothing else like it for years. As I headed out to run one last leg, I no longer wondered if I'd finish. The question now became, where would that finish line lead me?

For the next two miles, when the trail pitched toward the peaks, T. J. and I walked. When it flattened out, we ran. I was tired, but T. J. was deep in the hurt locker, and when the flat sections stretched out into some distance, a sizable gap opened between us. I'm not a chatty runner, so I thought he was giving me some space, but after I started walking again, he caught me, and his breath sounded heavy and jagged. When we hit the last two miles of Turquoise Lake, one of the last long, flat sections of the race, he could not hang.

The trail wrapped around the alpine lake, which was surrounded by craggy peaks, until it intersected with a steep jeep trail. A volunteer was stationed there in a van to guide exhausted runners in the proper direction. I was out of food and water, but that wasn't my concern when I asked the volunteer if he had anything to spare. The guy handed me one unwrapped Pop Tart. I thanked him and waited, holding that darn thing for ten minutes, then fifteen. A few runners passed me, but there was no sign of T. J., so I took off running…away from the finish line!

After half a mile, I saw T. J. walking my way. To say he was surprised to see me would be an understatement, and when I handed him that frosted snack, it sent him into a tailspin. As he ate, he lamented that he'd come to Colorado to support me, and now I was turning the tables to help get him to the finish line. He knew I'd abandoned my shot at a PR, saw me getting reeled in over and over, and felt like dead weight.

A few minutes later, sometime around two in the morning, we reached the van again and began navigating a steep decline beneath a starry sky. A couple of headlamps came bobbing up from behind, getting closer and closer. It was another runner and his pacer. The runner slowed down as he caught us. When he recognized me, he stopped and smiled. I thought he was just another friendly dude happy to be nearing the finish line, but he had something else on his mind.

"My son told me you were out here," he said. "He actually challenged me to catch you. And I guess I caught you."

"I guess you did," I said. He nodded, pleased with himself, and ran off.

"I can't believe that guy." T. J. shook his head as we watched him get swallowed by the night. "He didn't catch you!"

"Forget about him," I said. It bothered me too, but I didn't want T. J. to see that. It would only make him feel worse.

"If it weren't for me, he never would have even seen you." T. J.'s eyes flashed with the first signs of life I'd seen in miles. He was more annoyed than I was. "He didn't catch you. He caught your pacer!"

He was so angry, in fact, that he started to run for a stretch, then staggered and walked to catch his breath. That sequence played out a few times. It was pretty clear he couldn't maintain a workable pace, but that wasn't the point. T. J. was sending me a message. He knew I still had plenty in the tank and that crossing the finish line with any amount of unburned fuel is a cardinal sin. With his hands on his knees, he turned to me and said, "What are you still doing here? You need to go hunt that guy down!"

That was music to my ears. We shared an evil smile, and I took off. When I made the last turn on the racecourse, I had a gradual three-mile incline to hammer to reach the finish line. All but the elite of the elite walk that final stretch, which meant if I drained my tank, I would pass some runners. I had taken a snapshot of that smug dude in my mind's eye, and I wanted to catch him.

I used to take snapshots like that all the time. When I was a full-time savage, if you said something smart to me, I talked trash right back to you and used your disrespect as ammunition to propel me into whatever brutal task or race or workout I had lined up next. And there was always something.

We all have that ferocity—that dog—inside us. It's a natural response to provocation, a close cousin of the survival instinct, but most of us keep it chained up and locked away behind closed doors because that savage side of ourselves doesn't mix well with this "civilized" world. It's obsessive. It's always hungry, always looking for scraps of nourishment and finds them in competition, failure, and disrespect. I used to open that door on a regular basis, but as my life changed, I locked that beast away like almost everybody else and started letting those slights go. Any shade tossed in my direction was shed quicker than water down a duck's back. I'd matured and decided to live a more balanced life. That wasn't necessarily a bad thing, but it wasn't all good either.

I wasn't hungry anymore. I passed over a lot of juicy scraps for years, but that smug runner's casual comment did not slide down my back. The dog was hungry again, and on that agonizing final stretch, I realized how much I missed the feeling of being obsessed, the buzz I get from draining the tank dry. I'd deprived myself of it for way too long.

If you want to maximize minimal potential and become great in any field, you must embrace your savage side and become imbalanced, at least for a period of time. You'll need to funnel every minute of every single day into the pursuit of that degree, that starting spot, that job, that edge. Your mind must never leave the cockpit. Sleep at the library or the office. Hoop long past sundown and fall asleep watching film of your next opponent. There are no days off, and there is no downtime when you are obsessed with being great. That is what it takes to be the best ever at what you do.

Know that your dedication will be misunderstood. Some relationships may break down. The savage is not a socialized beast, and an imbalanced lifestyle often appears selfish from the outside. But the reason I've been able to help so many people with my life story is precisely because I embraced being that imbalanced while I pursued the impossible dream of becoming the hardest person ever. That's a mythical title, but it became my compass bearing, my North Star.

And there it was again, flickering in the Colorado sky, brighter than all the other galaxies. It guided me up that hill and into another flowing rhythm as I passed five more runners. Each headlamp I collected yielded more energy to burn, and with a mile and a half to go in the race, I reeled in my last one. It was that smug dude. I didn't approach on the far-left side of the gravel road. I rushed right up on his shoulder. I didn't touch him, but I was a hair's width from him because I didn't want him to be confused or disoriented in the darkness of night. I wanted him to know exactly who had run him down.

He had no clue that when he found me a few miles back, minding my own business, I was helping my pacer. He couldn't have known how much energy I had left, but when you don't know who it is you're talking to, the wise move is to lead with respect or say nothing at all. Instead, he ran his mouth, dropped some scraps, and fed the hungry dog inside me. Oh, but he had nothing to say when I blew past him. And neither did I. I didn't even give him the satisfaction of looking over, but I heard him huffing and puffing, and when he lowered his head in shame, I was reminded of why you should always beware of spitting in the wind.

I'd run a good race and finished in thirty-fifth place at 22:55:44, forty minutes slower than 2007 but still a darn good time considering there had been twelve long years and two heart surgeries between starts. Kish had never seen me finish a 100-miler. She was elated when I crossed the line and expected some big Hallmark moment, but I wasn't in the mood to celebrate. Like Colonel Trautman said about Rambo, "What you call hell, he calls home." And that's exactly what I felt when I crossed the line. That I'd finally made it back home.

But there was a storm brewing: the same borderline medical emergency that happens after every ultra race I finish, which meant we had to get back to our crew cabin in Breckenridge STAT. I stared out the window, fixated on my North Star as it tailed us on the forty-five-minute drive, tempting me to leave the soft life of balance and comfort behind and follow it. That told me that Leadville was not the one-off I had assumed it to be. Part of my hesitation in signing up in the first place was because I'd already done it. I'd run almost every meaningful race in the ultra game. I'd been there and done all of that, and now I knew that it wasn't enough!

What was next? Was it possible to operate as a full-time savage at forty-five years old, and if I gave it a shot, how long could I hold out? Those were questions for another night because before we pulled into the driveway, my body had already started to tighten up. I could feel the tremors coming on too, and while I knew what was next, this was unchartered territory for Kish.

The post-ultra unraveling was about to begin.

EVOLUTION NO. 4

lthough my childhood stuttering was alarming, I wasn't completely undone by trauma. I was distracted by toxic stress. My pain kept me from living a complete and happy life in grade school, and it continued to haunt me into young adulthood, yet through it all, I retained enough self-awareness to realize how bad things were and remember each and every corner I cut. Strange as it sounds, I was one of the lucky ones. For some victims, their trauma is so devastating that they lose all their self-respect and self-awareness. They are torn down to the studs. Foundational aspects of their character pounded to dust.

Part of what saved me from sliding all the way to rock bottom was what I saw in my mother. As much as she tried to hide it, she was the portrait of devastation. Which is why I've been able to study the work of the prisoner's mind all my life.

She'd been a young woman when she met Trunnis. He

dazzled her until she was spellbound. Then, with every slap to the face, every hateful, disrespectful comment, each time he cheated on her, he siphoned more of her life force away until she lost contact with the attractive, intelligent, dignified, strong woman she used to be. It didn't happen overnight. It rarely does. In abusive relationships, it's almost always gradual, which is why it burns so deep. Until one day, you wake up owned by the person who is destroying you.

In nature, destruction always gives way to creation, and my mother didn't sit in her rubble for long once we arrived in Indiana. An urge to build again is in each of us, and she had it too. However, when you are rebuilding the self, it must be done consciously. She'd lost all her confidence and emotional coherence because she never completely liberated herself from my father. As a result, she didn't know what she was building, and the bricks she laid became her prison cell. Subconsciously, she built a tower of mental and emotional isolation, and by the time I was eight years old, she was an empty shell. She hustled and strived, but very little registered with her emotionally. We lived parallel lives. I couldn't even reach her.

The irony is you build those walls to protect yourself. You think they will make you hard and less vulnerable, but they isolate you in solitary confinement with your darkest thoughts and ugliest memories. You convince yourself that somehow you deserve to be there due to the bad life decisions you made. You believe that you are not worthy of more, or something better, and that the damage can't be undone. You are filled with endless shame. When you look in the mirror, you don't see yourself for who you are. And what keeps you locked up in your prison is that false narrative that you continually feed yourself and the false reflection you can't escape because it is part of you. By the time I was in high school, my mom was an independent, successful woman who had survived domestic violence and landed a six-figure job at a top-tier liberal arts university. Those were the straight facts. Everyone around us saw the same thing, but in the mirror, she saw a worthless and undeserving person.

While working as a college dean during my junior year of high school, she volunteered as a teacher in a prison. It wasn't enough for her to be in her own mental prison; she wanted to experience a real one. Especially if it meant she'd have less time to sit with herself and consider her life in any meaningful way. After just a few weeks of work at the penitentiary, her daily routine—which had been damn near sacred since we arrived in Indiana—was all over the place, and I sensed something was off. How could I not, with the phone ringing every fifteen minutes? Weeks before I was to leave for Air Force boot camp, she finally explained what was going on. She was engaged to a man who'd been in a maximum-security prison for the last ten years.

It took more than a few minutes for that statement to register before I asked, "What was he in prison for?" She didn't answer right away. She had to collect her thoughts because there is no easy way of telling your son that your future husband is in prison for murdering a woman over drugs. He didn't shoot her. This wasn't an attempted robbery gone wrong. This man straight-up choked the life out of a woman over drugs. She went on to say that he was due to be released from prison the week after I left for boot camp and would be moving into our house.

It is truly amazing what the mind can do when you fail to rebuild yourself consciously. My dad was a gangster and a crook. Her previous fiancé had been murdered in his own garage, and for an encore, she would marry a convicted murderer less than a week after his release from prison. My mom was looking for someone she could save because she did not have the strength to save herself. But the marriage did not go well. They would divorce within two years. He would relapse and eventually die of an overdose many years later.

To put it into plain text: when your self-worth goes away and you don't deal with or accept your demons, they will continue to own you, and you will become a bottom feeder.

I'm aware that most of the advice I give and stories I tell are built to help you push through impossible situations. However, sometimes what you need is a Hard Stop. If you ever find yourself in an abusive scenario like my mother's or any sort of battle where you are losing your sense of self and verging on erasure, your best hope is to arrest the slide before you hit rock bottom.

Hard Stops allow military units and individual soldiers to reorg. That includes reloading your empty magazines, taking inventory of your ammunition, and rearranging your gear so you have access to loaded weapons and anything else you may need in the hours ahead. You also must take a hard look at your battle plan and get a clear sense of what it is you're facing and where it will lead.

I know firsthand how torturous it is to be continually stalked by a predator. You lose all sense of normalcy. Reality becomes distorted, but I also know that moments of clarity do exist. My mom should have reorg'd after Trunnis smacked her in the face the first time, or the twelfth time, or even the fiftieth time. While I know this is hard to do, it is something that we must do for ourselves. It is non-negotiable. If she had, she might have noticed she was on a slippery slope that would lead to her utter destruction. She may have seen that it was not normal or tolerable to watch her kids work all-night skates day after day and then get beaten at home. In a toxic situation, you cannot keep moving blindly forward hoping it will end. It won't, but you might.

When you arrest the slide, you will be damaged but not completely broken. Your wound will likely become a distraction, but with intention and effort, you can heal and take control of your life. When you come to at rock bottom, that's a different situation, and it won't be a clean or easy fix. When inmates are released, they generally aren't rehabilitated in a sustainable way. Most leave prison jacked up and often need more help if they are to piece their lives back together. You'll need help too. You'll need to find people who have survived or at least relate to what you've been through and can help you heal.

Of course, it takes self-esteem and self-awareness to seek help and share your brutal story, and when you are confined by the walls you built, awareness and confidence are non-existent. At that point, your only choice is to get angry.

We are too often told that anger is an unhealthy emotion, but when someone or something has stolen your soul and destroyed your life, anger is a natural response. I am not talking about irrational rage, which can be disastrous and lead you down an even darker hole. I am talking about controlled anger, which is a natural source of energy that can wake you up and help you realize that what you went through wasn't right. I have cracked open anger several times. It has warmed me when I was freezing, it has turned my fear into bravery, and it has given me fight when I had none. And it can do the same for you.

Anger will snap you out of the spell you're in until you are no longer willing to remain confined in your mental prison. You'll be scratching and clawing at the walls, looking for cracks where the light leaks in. Your fingernails will be broken, the tips of your fingers bloody and raw, and you will continue to fight to expand those cracks because your anger will be purifying and the human mind loves progress. Keep at it, and eventually, those walls will tumble until you are free, standing in a debris field one more time, with your eyes wide open. That'll work. Because destruction always breeds creation.

> Have the courage and mental endurance to do whatever it takes to start knocking down those walls. You are the warden of your life. Don't forget you hold the keys. #PrisonerMind #NeverFinished

CHAPTER FIVE

DISCIPLE OF DISCIPLINE

My vision narrowed as we pulled into the driveway at the crew cabin in Breckenridge, Colorado. It was just after four in the morning and pitch-black. I could barely see as I stepped carefully down the short staircase leading to the front door. Kish watched me, concerned, as I entered the house under my own power. I was hurting but holding it together, and she knew I wouldn't show any weakness in front of my team. In fact, she assumed I'd keep walking all the way through our bedroom on the ground floor and into the bathroom where she could help me get undressed and cleaned up. But the thin thread I'd been gripping tight to remain upright and presentable was fraying fast, and as soon as the guys were out of sight, it snapped. My knees buckled, and I fell to the bedroom floor.

Kish was right behind me. She closed the door and locked it, ripped the cover off the bed, and spread it on the floor beside me. Then did her best to reposition me onto the bedspread to give me some semblance of comfort. She had no clue that her attentiveness made me anything but comfortable.

Kish is such a neat freak she is borderline OCD. Dust, dirt, and the potential for germs get her radar pinging on high alert. She's the first to comment when there is something foul in the air, and here I was smelling like an old dog who had rolled in roadkill. My legs and feet were covered in mud and blood, my fingernails rimmed with dirt. A paste of filth and sweat coated my skin from toe to scalp. My breath was rapid, rancid, and shallow, and the mild tremors that had only been visible to Kish in the car because she was paying close attention had become bone-rattling shivers. Then, my bowels groaned, and I knew it was about to get a whole lot worse.

This was nothing new for me. Ever since my first ultra, the San Diego One Day, the aftermath of every 100-mile race I'd completed included a tidal wave of pain and suffering, along with a humiliating loss of control of my most basic bodily functions. Kish knew that, but she had never experienced it firsthand, and I was nervous she wouldn't be able to handle it.

The two of us are very different people. Kish is not the outdoorsy type. If it weren't for me, she never would have heard of Leadville. Her idea of fun is spending the day on a pickleball court or golf course or chilling at a five-star resort. She's prissy. I'm a holdover beast from a different age, but when it comes to hard work and discipline, that's where we marry up. She keeps up in the gym and on the roads and trails, is a hard-charger when it comes to business, and understands my dedication to the grind in a way that no other woman—no other person—in my life ever has.

Yet, aside from that one night in the Nashville ER, she'd only ever seen me as capable of enduring and withstanding almost anything and everything with little to no help, and often on very little sleep. I'd rarely shown her any vulnerability, so how would she feel about me once she saw I wasn't even capable of wiping myself? Ashamed and embarrassed, I told her what was about to go down, and she looked horrified.

"Wait, David! Not on the duvet!"

"The what?" I asked, delirious.

"The duvet." I must have looked confused because I'd never heard the word "duvet" in my entire life. "You know, the comforter goes inside the duvet." Kish looked frazzled as she shook the snow-white linen beneath me, which, to her abject horror, was getting soaked through with my foul post-race marinade. "You're lying on it right now!"

"You mean the blanket?" I asked. She dashed out of the room without answering and returned with a black trash bag that she spread between me and the precious duvet like an open diaper. Only then did she tug my running shorts down to my thighs. My bowels unclenched, and an ungodly stench rose up around us.

As predicted, she had to wipe my behind because I couldn't move, and then she helped me up onto my knees so I could piss into some high-end decorative glass fruit bowl she'd found upstairs in the kitchen while she clenched her teeth and stressed about what this might do to her Airbnb rating.

After all of that, after she'd peeled the shoes and socks off my feet, cleaned me up the best she could, and cocooned me in that ridiculous duvet, my eyes rolled up behind my sagging eyelids. I wasn't sleeping. I was attempting to savor the uncontrollable shivers, the filth, my own sick stench, and the many flavors of pain.

The crushing agony in my hip flexors was searing. The only other time I'd ever felt anything like that was during the Wednesday night of my second Hell Week when I was rousted after a five-minute power nap on the beach. Everyone else on my boat crew was getting a full hour, but not me. Psycho Pete, the instructor I hated the most, wanted a private audience. I remember trying to stand up with that maniac in my face. It felt like my hips were trapped in a vice. The only thing that would have eased the throb was curling up in the fetal position, so that's what I did in Breckenridge, tripping on how pain has the power to bring you back in time like nothing else. As I lay there, shivering and sweating at the same time, I could have sworn I was back on Coronado Island, getting wet and sandy.

Kish was terrified. She watched me, timed my arrhythmic breaths, and listened to my bones rattle as she mapped out emergency contingencies in her head. Was I in shock? Was I having some sort of altitude reaction? Breckenridge is at 9,600 feet. She was concerned my condition could deteriorate fast. But I wasn't worried about any of that. I knew that this was my old friend, breakdown. My final phase of ultra.

When I first got into endurance events, I loved the break-down phase because the suffering made me feel alive and reminded me that I'd gone all-out. This time, I didn't relish it in the same way, but I knew that breakdown was a byproduct of an all-out effort and that if I explored the crevices of my mind, I would find valuable lessons, which tend to spill out with any unraveling. Most people prefer to avoid breakdowns like this because the suffering can be so overwhelming, it just might mark you forever. I embrace breakdown and welcome the scarring. There is a lot of information in scar tissue.

Scars are proof that the past is real. Physical scars never go away, and when you look at them, they can bring you right back to a specific place in time. But the scar tissue that builds up around that old injury is weak. Professional fighters who've been hit in the face thousands of times bleed faster than those who have never been punched. Once you've been cut deep, you are forever vulnerable to bleeding.

The same is true for the mental and emotional scars that we all carry with us, the scars we cannot see. They might be invisible, but they affect us much more severely than physical scars. Mental and emotional scars are our weak spots, and they can open up just as easily as physical scars unless we do the work to strengthen them. If you haven't dealt with your scars, they can alter your life's path. You will be prone to failure during difficult physical and emotional situations, whether that's during an athletic event, at work, or in your home life, and eventually, you will land back in front of your mirror that never lies.

Breakdown is its own kind of mirror. Whatever you're made of is laid out in front of you clear and plain. Your history and mindset become a weathered old map ridged with your scars, and if you read them like an archeologist on a dig, you might uncover the code you need to rise again and become better and stronger. Because there is no transformation without breakdown, and there is always another evolution, another skin to shed, a better or deeper version of ourselves waiting to be revealed.

I did a quick inventory of my scars as I faded into that slippery headspace between waking and dreaming. Psycho Pete's voice trailed off, and another familiar yet faint voice that I couldn't quite place called out to me.

"David, wake up…" My memory convulsed and bled into my reality, and I couldn't tell where I was or what was real. "David," he said, gruffly, louder this time. "Time to get up, boy!"

It was the voice of my grandfather Sergeant Jack Gardner. Unlike those who embrace affectionate nicknames like Pop-Pop, Poppa, or Grandpa, he'd instructed me to call him Sgt. Jack, and that set the tone for how things were going to be between us. Oh yes, he left more than a few scars etched in my brain, and he was shaking me awake just like old times.

❀ ❀ ❀

It was the summer of 1983 when we staggered up his long gravel driveway and arrived on his doorstep under-slept, underfed, and with all our possessions crammed into black trash bags. My mother knocked on the door. While we waited, I scanned the yard. My grandparents had a big property—a full acre of land—including a wide, perfectly manicured lawn with train tracks running along one side. There wasn't a blade of green grass out of place and not a single weed in sight. That should have been my first warning.

While my dad was convinced that my grandparents had been behind our escape from Buffalo, he didn't witness our arrival or my grandmother Morna's wordless greeting on the front porch. She opened the door, rolled her eyes, and waved us inside. Sgt. Jack stood behind her with the expression of a drill instructor watching new recruits get off the bus with their long hair and beards, all wet behind the ears. He'd been a master sergeant in the Air Force and had retired years ago but was dressed in one of his flight suits. I didn't recognize the look on his face because I was a disoriented young pup all covered in scar tissue, but when I went to boot camp for the first time, I saw it again. That day in Brazil, though, he looked like a hero to me. I smiled. He did not smile back.

It felt good to be there anyway. I was happy to be anywhere but on Paradise Road, and they were relieved that we'd all gotten away from my father, but that didn't mean room, board, and babysitting would be free. The first bill came due before dawn the next morning when I was awakened by a stiff shake of my shoulders. I opened my eyes, and there was Sgt. Jack, still in uniform.

"Time to get up, boy," he said. "There's work to do." I wiped my eyes and glanced at my brother, who shrugged. It was still dark outside, we were exhausted from the trip, and as soon as Sgt. Jack left the room, we fell back to sleep. The next wake-up call came in the form of glasses of cold water thrown in our faces. Two minutes later, we were in the garage where he kept his old metal desk from the military. On the corner of that desk was a yellow note pad. The top of the page was titled "Task List," dated and marked "0530." I had no clue what those numbers meant until Sgt. Jack explained that his house ran on military time.

That was the moment I realized that there would be no adjustment period and no coddling whatsoever. My grandparents never expressed basic sympathy for what we had been through. Sgt. Jack simply stared hard, went over the list, and walked us through the garage as if we were his new employees and needed to know where to find the rakes, hoes, hedge clippers, and his quiver of brooms and dustpans and how to operate and clean his manual lawn mower. He didn't care how we divided up the work, just that we got up and got to it on time. Each day started like that. With an unwelcome wake-up call, an itemized, military-time-stamped task list, and few, if any, words from the old man.

Sgt. Jack was half Black and half Native American, and though he was only five-foot-seven, he had a larger presence about him. He'd worked as a cook in the Air Force and still dressed in military attire every day. It was usually a flight suit or one of his Battle Dress Uniforms on weekdays. His crisp Dress Blues were reserved for church and all other formal occasions. Sgt. Jack took great pride in detailed stewardship. He cared about everything he owned. He had two separate two-car garages and four cars on the property, Cadillacs and Chevrolets from the midcentury. Like his well-tended house and garden, those cars were pristine.

Born in 1905, he came of age in Southern Indiana during the height of Jim Crow, when it was dangerous to be a Black man in America and a wrong word or look could spark a lynch mob. His parents were poor, and he wasn't babied as a kid. His formal education ended in the fourth grade when he had to get a job to help support the family. So, when I landed in his house, he passed along what he'd learned. What they'd taught him worked as far as he was concerned. He had a military pension. He owned his house free and clear, same with every car in his garages, and he had money in the bank. Sgt. Jack was squared away, and he got there with a self-reliance on detail and discipline.

Each morning, before he woke me up, he walked the perimeter of his property, surveying the lawn, several trees, and the long unpaved driveway blanketed in snow-white gravel. The house had two porches, one on either side, and he liked them swept and his rain gutters cleared of debris at all times because storms come down hard in that part of the country. Sgt. Jack couldn't stand seeing leaf litter, dust, or weeds. Everything had to be immaculate.

The daily task list was always at least ten tasks long. Sometimes, it stretched to over twenty. The first order of business in the morning was to sweep both porches, front and back. After that, I had to get out the rake and collect and bag any stray leaves that had fallen overnight. In the spring and summer, that wasn't a huge job, but in the fall, when the leaves turned, it took hours.

Hedges and grass grew like crazy during the humid Indiana summer, and that meant mowing the lawn manually in a perfect grid and clipping all the hedges almost daily. Weeds were always a problem in the summer, and as soon as they began poking through the gravel on the driveway, I had to get on my hands and knees and dig into the dirt to pull the roots free. The gravel dug into my skin, leaving scrapes and bruises. To me, it didn't feel a whole lot different from scraping gum off the skate-rink floor at first. In those early weeks, I took Sgt. Jack's tasks as a sign that no matter where I lived or who I lived with, I was bound to suffer at the hands of a bully. My scarred young mind was deep in the woe-is-me rinse cycle.

So was my brother's. He didn't last long on Sgt. Jack detail and retreated to Buffalo pretty quickly. Crazy to think that Buffalo seemed like the better option. I wasn't going anywhere, but that doesn't mean I enjoyed it. At first, I despised the man and attempted to rebel. He'd come shake me awake, and I wouldn't move. Then he'd splash water in my face, and I took that too. If I still didn't get up, he'd come to my bedside with a metal trash can lid and whack it with a wooden spoon right next to my ear until I was up and on my way to the garage to pick up my orders.

I didn't yet realize that Sgt. Jack was no Trunnis. He was my Mr. Miyagi. Not in the sense that each chore came with specific instructions or that those instructions would manifest in skills that would deliver karate-tournament salvation. He never sat back and said, "I'm teaching you how to be a responsible young man." Yet, I learned valuable life lessons.

Many of us will meet people like Sgt. Jack in our lives, an elder or teacher who refuses to tell us what we want to hear in the way we want to hear it. When you're emotionally scarred like I was, any and every hard look or gruff reply, any order or mandate, can feel like a personal attack, and oftentimes, we tune them out to our own detriment. It took me a long time to understand that there wasn't anything personal about Sgt. Jack's approach or his list. It was all transactional.

His daughter—my mother—needed a place for us to stay, and in the real world, lodging isn't free. As far as Sgt. Jack was concerned, that daily task list was the nightly bill to be paid. Not that my mom gave it a second thought. She was busy with a full load of classes at the local university and two part-time jobs, a schedule she'd keep for the next six years until she graduated with a master's degree. The bill would have to be paid in my sweat.

Once school started, my work was divided into before- and after-school sessions, and there was rarely any respite. After I got home, schoolwork came first. Then, I had to complete all the tasks on the list correctly before I was allowed to play basketball with my friends. At first, I had no idea what doing a particular task correctly meant to the old man. The only direct feedback I got from him was a straight-faced nod, which meant he approved, or a shake of the head, which meant, "Try again."

I saw that a lot. His head shake of doom stalked me into my nightmares, where I would mow a lawn that never stopped growing out of control or attempt to clear rain gutters that were rimmed with saw-toothed blades that threatened to chop my fingers off.

All things being equal, I preferred to be outside. I considered most of the house a no-go zone because as badly as I felt I was being treated by Sgt. Jack, I much preferred him to Morna. She was also of mixed race and could pass for White if or when she needed to. She celebrated that fact by spraying the N-word around like an Ecolab exterminator hunting for a hive of cockroaches. More often than not, her favorite word landed on my head. For all the racists I met in Brazil, nobody called me "nigger" more than sweet grandma Morna, which only heightened the feeling that I was their personal slave.

Months passed, and the tyranny did not relent. By then, I knew exactly what Sgt. Jack expected from me. I knew how to cut the grass, rake the leaves, and wash the cars the way he wanted, but I felt sorry for myself because few, if any, of my friends had to do chores at all, let alone complete a daily, military-grade task list. Plus, my grandparents still hadn't demonstrated any empathy for what I'd been through during the first eight years of my life.

Clearly, they didn't understand me. I was housed in their guestroom with dated furniture and wallpaper. I didn't have basketball posters on the walls. I wasn't given toys or cool sneakers or a stereo. Did they put out any effort to make that room more accommodating for a kid? No chance! And the only way I could get back at them was by doing a half-hearted job instead of working hard on the all-important tasks of the day. Of course, I was only victimizing myself.

If I wasn't done before dinnertime, they'd call me in. The meals were not kid-friendly. There were no burgers or hot dogs. It was baked chicken or roast meats with sides of collard greens, chitlins, and cabbage. I was expected to clean my plate, whether I liked the food or not, and then go back out and finish whichever tasks remained undone. I often worked well past sundown.

I couldn't understand why my grandparents treated me this

way. The only explanation my jacked-up eight-year-old brain could find was that, like my father, they hated me and resented my presence in their home. Which is why in the early days, earning Sgt. Jack's checkmark of approval meant nothing to me, and I sleepwalked through his tasks like a zombie. I figured any attempt was good enough. *Screw it, and screw him*, I thought. I hated the old man and didn't care what he thought of me.

Six months later, though I still loathed the man, I changed my approach to the task list. I got up after the first wake-up call without delay. There would be no more early-morning baptisms for me. Instead, I focused on the details Sgt. Jack always noticed and finished each job right the first time. That was the only way I'd get any free time to play basketball. However, my new approach produced an unexpected side effect as well: a sense of pride in a job well done. In fact, that sense of pride came to mean more to me than basketball time.

When I washed his car collection, a weekly assignment, I knew every drop of water had to be wiped away with a chamois before the first coat of wax. I used SOS pads to get the white walls gleaming and buffed out every panel. I also used Armor All on the dashboards and all the vinyl insides. I buffed the leather seats too. It bothered me if I saw streaks on the glass or chrome. I was annoyed if I missed a soiled spot or cut a corner here or there on any chore. I didn't know it at the time, but that was a sign that I was actually healing.

When a half-hearted job doesn't bother you, it speaks volumes about the kind of person you are. And until you start feeling a sense of pride and self-respect in the work you do, no matter how small or overlooked those jobs might be, you will continue to sell yourself short. I knew I had every reason in the world to rebel and remain lazy. I also sensed that would only make me more miserable, so I adapted. But no matter how well I did or how fast I completed a given task, there were no atta' boys or weekly allowance. No ice cream cones or surprise gifts, hugs, or high fives. In Sgt. Jack's mind, I was finally doing what I should have been doing all along.

My grandparents weren't ice-cold to everyone. When my cousin came to stay for Christmas in 1983, there were hugs and kisses aplenty from both Morna and Sgt. Jack because, unlike my mother, his mom insisted they treat her child with affection, not military discipline. The gifts piled up too. There were toys and clothes and a barbecue where burgers and hot dogs were grilled to order, followed by bowls full of ice cream. Whatever he wanted and whenever he wanted it, my cousin got it.

"David, come on over here for a minute," Sgt. Jack said while I eyeballed my cousin Damien as he scarfed down his bowl of ice cream. He'd been there for two days and had enjoyed more ice cream than I had in six months. "I have a gift for you too."

I followed him, almost shocked, until it became clear we were headed out into the garage as usual. Evidently, it was time to find out what a Christmas-morning task list looked like. Christmas was no different than the average Wednesday to my grandfather. He didn't care if it was your birthday or any other holiday. The work would not stop. I grabbed the sheet of paper off his desk as he wheeled over my Christmas present. It was a shiny new manual lawnmower with my initials monogrammed on the gleaming stainless-steel wheel hubs. There was snow on the ground, so I knew I didn't need to mow the lawn that morning, but there had been a sale on yard equipment at Western Auto, and the old man never could pass up a sale.

"Merry Christmas," he said with a grin. My cousin was being treated like a prince, and the old man brought me out to the garage to troll me. I guess I've had a lot of Merry Christmases in my life.

Two separate events would soon change how I saw Sgt. Jack forever. In the new year, my mom and I moved into our subsidized seven-dollar-a-month apartment in Lamplight Manor. The following summer, she enrolled me in summer school down the road. One day, after class let out, I walked home with a group of kids who lived nearby. One of them, a little girl named Meredith, lived down the street, and we covered the last stretch together. Her father happened to be sitting on their front porch drinking a beer when we got to her house, and as soon as he saw me, he put that beer down, leaned forward, stroked his beard, and glared at me like a mad dog.

Mind you, while my grandmother called me the N-word, I had never experienced any racism in public before. I simply thought he was mad at his daughter when he barked, "Meredith, get inside!" I didn't think his stress had anything to do with me. Later that evening, he called my mom and warned her that he was in the Ku Klux Klan.

"Tell your son to leave my daughter alone," he said.

After she told him to go to hell, he said he would pay Sgt. Jack a visit. Everyone knew Sgt. Jack in Brazil, Indiana. He was friends with the mayor and other local leaders, who all considered him to be a churchgoing patriot, a man of God and his word. He was proof that the American Dream was real, and in the minds of many racist White boys in Brazil, he was one of "the good ones." Clearly, this fool thought Sgt. Jack would straighten her and me out. My mom smiled at the thought.

"Please do," she said. Then she hung up and called her father.

When I saw Meredith's dad again a few days later, he was on my grandparents' front porch. He'd come by unannounced, but Sgt. Jack was prepared. He looped his pistol through his belt and wore it like a sidearm when he opened his front door. I was huddled inside behind my grandfather and around a corner but had a clear view when Meredith's father noticed Sgt. Jack's weapon and backed up a step. Sgt. Jack raised his chin another inch, looked the man dead in the eye, but didn't say a word.

"Look, Jack," the Klansman began, "if your grandson doesn't stop walking home from school with my daughter, we are going to have some problems."

"The only problem we're gonna have," Sgt. Jack said, "is a dead Klansman on my front porch if you don't get off my property."

I ran to the door in time to watch that man turn around, get back in his truck, and drive off. Then I looked over at Sgt. Jack, who nodded. It was the first time any adult had protected me from harm.

A few months later, I was in the driveway with Sgt. Jack and his friend Bill while they worked on my grandfather's Cadillac. Those two tinkered with cars almost every day. If they weren't changing spark plugs or checking oil, Sgt. Jack was flushing a radiator or steam cleaning an engine. When the day's job was done, Bill slammed the steel hood down without realizing Sgt. Jack's hands were still resting on the rim. The hood shattered fingers on both of his hands, but he didn't make a sound.

"Bill, lift the hood," he said, calmly, still in complete control. The blood drained from Bill's face when he realized what he'd done. He was so shook, it took a few seconds for him to jiggle the hood's release. When he finally got it, Sgt. Jack pulled his bloody hands free, walked calmly into the house, and found my grandmother.

"Morna," he said, "I think you'd better drive me to the hospital."

Witnessing that changed me. I'd never been around such strength and composure. I didn't even know something like that was possible, and I thought if I could be as tough as him one day, all of the suffering at the hands of my father, the shoveling snow and gravel, the raking leaves and washing cars, the cleaning rain gutters, the clipping hedges, and the lawn mowing would be worth it. I was still struggling to learn, to trust, to feel good about myself, and to find meaning in all the pain, but by seeing how Sgt. Jack handled that situation, I learned that being tough could be my way out.

I don't mean my way out of Brazil. That wasn't top of mind yet. I was looking for a way out of my fragile, wounded state of mind. There's an old saying in the military, that "if you are stupid, you better be hard." Back then, I considered myself stupid. Partly because all that scar tissue was still so fresh it was hard to focus on my schoolwork, and my response was simply to be lazy. If I failed because I didn't try, did I really fail? Then, I learned to cheat my way through. Sgt. Jack's way didn't involve whining, scheming, or feeling sorry for yourself. He was about gritting his teeth, taking pride in everything he did, and dealing head-on with whatever came his way.

For longer than I could remember, I'd felt neglected and ignored. I was bitter when my friends and cousin could play when they wanted to, watch television all day, and wear fresh gear to school. When would I ever get mine, I wondered? When would I get something for me and me alone? That day in the driveway was when I finally figured out that Sgt. Jack's example was the gift I'd been hoping for all along. It was more impressive and satisfying than any present could be, tastier than any hamburger or hot dog, and sweeter than an ice cream sundae. It was the best and most important day in my miserable life so far.

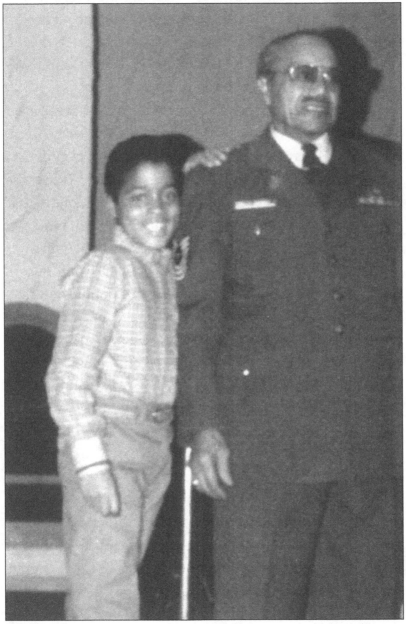

With my Mr. Miyagi

Sgt. Jack was a hard teacher, but kids need hard teachers sometimes. I know that might hurt your ears because things are different now. We are warned of the lasting effects of stress on children, and to compensate, parents strategize about how to make their children's lives comfortable and easy. But is the real world always comfortable? Is it easy? Life is not G-rated. We must prepare kids for the world as it is.

Our generation is training kids to become full-fledged members of Entitlement Nation, which ultimately makes them easy prey for the lions among us. Our ever-softening society doesn't just affect children. Adults fall into the same trap. Even those of us who have achieved great things. Every single one of us is just another frog in the soon-to-be-boiling water that is our soft culture. We take unforeseen obstacles personally. We are ready to be outraged at all times by the evil ways of the world. Believe me, I know all about evil and have dealt with more of it than most, but if you catalog your scars to use them as excuses or a bargaining chip to make life easier for yourself, you've missed an opportunity to become better and grow stronger. Sgt. Jack knew what awaited me as an adult. He was preparing me for the grip of life. Whether he knew it or not, the man was training me to be a savage.

The evolutionary equation is the exact same for everybody. It doesn't matter who you are. You could be a young person looking to tap into your power and become great or a mid-life adult or senior who's never done a darn thing but wants to achieve something before it's too late. Or maybe you've achieved a lot but are overcoming injury or illness or are simply uninspired and caught in emotional and physical quicksand. First, you must recognize that you have fallen off or are perpetually falling short. Next, accept that you are on your own. Nobody will come save you. They may show you an example, like Sgt. Jack did for me and I'm doing for you right now, but it will be up to you to do the work. Then, you must become a disciple of discipline.

Even after we moved into our own place, whenever my mom had to work late or go out of town, I'd spend the night at Sgt. Jack's, and sure enough, there would be a wake-up call and a bill in the morning in the form of a task list. And yes, like my dad, Sgt. Jack was a mean old man who expected me to do as he said and work for free, but unlike Trunnis, he wrapped something valuable in the discipline he served, and whenever I put maximum focus to each task, I earned a sense of pride that I hadn't been able to find anyplace else.

But it didn't last.

Eventually, I grew into a rebellious teenager. I sagged my pants down, flipped the middle finger at authority, and was well on my way to flunking out. I had become a punk, but Sgt. Jack didn't try to tell me how to dress or act, beyond insisting that, when I come across an adult, I had better greet them with "sir" and "ma'am." And though he knew about each and every racial taunt and episode of vandalism I endured, he had no intention of stepping in to fight my battles anymore. I was almost grown, and they were my storms to navigate. Not his.

Like many disaffected teenagers, I wasn't living a mission-driven life. I was merely existing. I had become lazy, and my attention to detail was long gone because I didn't have that guy looking over my shoulder on a daily basis to keep me on point. The feeling of pride that I had back in the day working Sgt. Jack's property was nowhere to be found, but nobody considered this to be any kind of emergency. I was only seventeen, and even then, it was normal to give young kids plenty of space to do a whole lot of nothing much. We've all heard parents say, "He is only a teenager," or, "She's only in college," when explaining away bad habits or poor choices. The question is, when is the right time to start living instead of merely existing?

My time came when I received a letter informing me that my failing grades would keep me from graduating high school, which would also end my career in the Air Force before it started. The next day, I went back to Sgt. Jack and began staying over at his place more often. I asked for his task lists. I wanted to work in his yard. I craved discipline because I had a sense it might save me.

That's the beauty of discipline. It trumps everything. A lot of us are born with minimal talent, unhappy in our own skin and with the genetic makeup with which we were born. We have messed-up parents, grow up bullied and abused, or are diagnosed with learning disabilities. We hate our hometown, our teachers, our families, and nearly everything about ourselves. We wish we could be born again as someone else in some other time and place. Well, I am proof that rebirth is possible through discipline, which is the only thing capable of altering your DNA. It is the skeleton key that can get you past all the gatekeepers and into each and every room you wish to enter. Even the ones built to keep you out!

It's so easy to be great nowadays because so many people are focused on efficiency: getting the most for themselves with the least amount of time and effort. Let all of them leave the gym early, skip school, take sick days. Commit to becoming the one person with a never-ending task list.

This is where you make up the difference in potential. By learning to maximize what you do have, you will not only level the playing field but also surpass those born with more natural ability and advantages than you. Let your hours become days, then weeks, then years of effort. Allow discipline to seep into your cells until work becomes a reflex as automatic as breathing. With discipline as your medium, your life will become a work of art.

Discipline builds mental endurance because when effort is your main priority, you stop looking for everything to be enjoyable. Our phones and social media have turned too many of us inside out with envy and greed as we get inundated with other people's success, their new cars and houses, big contracts, resort vacations, and romantic getaways. We see how much fun everyone else is having and feel like the world is passing us by, so we complain about it and then wonder why we are not where we want to be.

When you become disciplined, you don't have time for that. Your insecurities become alarm bells reminding you that doing your chores or homework to the utmost of your ability and putting in extra time on the job or in the gym are requirements for a life well-lived. A drive for self-optimization and daily repetition will build your capacity for work and give you confidence that you can take on more. With discipline as your engine, your workload and output will double, then triple. What you won't see, at least not at first, is the fact that your own personal evolution has begun to bear fruit. You won't see it because you'll be too busy taking action.

Discipline does not have a belief system. It transcends class, color, and gender. It cuts through all the noise and strife. If you think that you are behind the eight ball for whatever reason, discipline is the great equalizer. It erases all disadvantages. Nowadays, it doesn't matter where you are from or who you are; if you are disciplined, there will be no stopping you.

Believe me, I know none of that comes easy. I struggled to get up before the sun on that first morning back on Sgt. Jack detail. I hadn't dealt with a 0500 wake-up call in so long, it felt too sudden. I was lethargic as the bed sucked me back into its cushy arms. The pull to stay lazy was stronger than it had ever been.

That's how it works when you're trying to change. The call to remain complacent will only grow louder until you silence it with a pattern of behavior that leaves no doubt about your mission. Lucky for me, I knew the stakes were too high to fall into that trap, so high that I didn't have time to wake up slowly. I needed to knock out my chores before school so I could hit the books after I got home.

Still drowsy and dragging, I remembered that whenever I ran or played ball, I felt better afterward. I was just a dumb kid. I didn't know anything about the science of endorphins and how they trigger an energized and positive feeling in the body and brain after a workout. But I knew how I felt, and that was enough. I dropped down and hit a max set of push-ups. By the time I was done, I had the energy I needed to run to the garage, grab my task list, and get to work. That became my new pattern. Wake up earlier than I had to, do my max set of push-ups, and then get cracking.

It was during those days of struggle and striving, when I didn't know if I would actually graduate or be accepted by the Air Force, that I first realized I am at my best when I am a disciple of discipline. The further I got away from it, and from Sgt. Jack, the worse I became. While I still didn't like waking up early or most of the chores I had to do, those were the very things that turned me into someone I could be proud of.

I also knew Sgt. Jack wouldn't always be around to lead by

example. He was already in his late eighties and had started to slow down. Old age had crept up on him. He slept much more and didn't move very well, which meant it was time to learn how to hold myself accountable. His task lists had taught me how to prioritize and attack each day with a plan of action, so I started getting up before him. I'd do my push-ups, walk the perimeter of his property well before dawn, and assess what needed to be done. By the time he was at his desk sipping coffee, I was already working.

Once he saw that I took the initiative to not only do the tasks that would normally be on the list but identify additional work to be done, his lists shrank and then disappeared altogether. At home, Sgt. Jack's task lists evolved into my Accountability Mirror, which helped me build the habits necessary to graduate on time, pass the ASVAB, and enlist in the Air Force.

From then on, whenever I had a purpose or a task in front of me, I didn't consider it done until I'd completed it to the best of my ability. When that's the way you live your life, you no longer need a task list or an Accountability Mirror because when you see the grass is high, you cut the grass right then. If you're lagging behind in school or work, you study harder or stay late and take care of business. When it came time to lose one hundred pounds to become a SEAL, I knew exactly what I had to do. I had to tap back into being a disciple of discipline, but I didn't need a task list. Writing it down would have only cut into my workout time, and I didn't have a single minute to spare.

Once, those task lists were a burden. Today, I burn with an inner drive shaped by doing the things I didn't want to do over and over again. And it won't let me relax until I've done what needs to be done every day.

My post-Leadville breakdown was physically challenging

yet mentally exhilarating because it allowed me to bask in the power of my mind. The hard work it took to get back to the starting line of Leadville demanded that I go back to being the disciple of discipline Sgt. Jack helped create. Granted, I still don't know what his objective was. Was he trying to shine a path forward and make me better, or did he just want free labor? In the end, it didn't matter. It was up to me to interpret why he did it, what it meant, and spin it to create forward momentum.

It will always be up to you to find the lesson in every challenging situation and use it to become stronger, wiser, and better. No matter what comes down on your head, you must find a glimmer of light, remain positive, and never treat yourself as a victim. Especially if you intend to thrive in a harsh world where you have to work for everything that matters. I'm not talking about material things. I'm talking about self-respect, self-love, and self-mastery.

Minutes before waking up to the morning after Leadville, rank as could be, with my foul shorts still looped around my thighs, I flashed to one of the last times I saw Sgt. Jack alive. It was at my graduation from basic training in the Air Force. In spite of his poor health, he was adamant about attending, and as a World War II vet, he was given a VIP seat on the dais among the brass.

All the years I knew him, he'd never said, "Good job," to me. I never once heard him say, "I love you." But when they announced my name and I marched across that stage in my Dress Blues to officially become an airman like him, we locked eyes, and I watched one solitary tear snake down his cheek. Sgt. Jack was beaming, and it was obvious that he was proud as hell to be my grandfather.

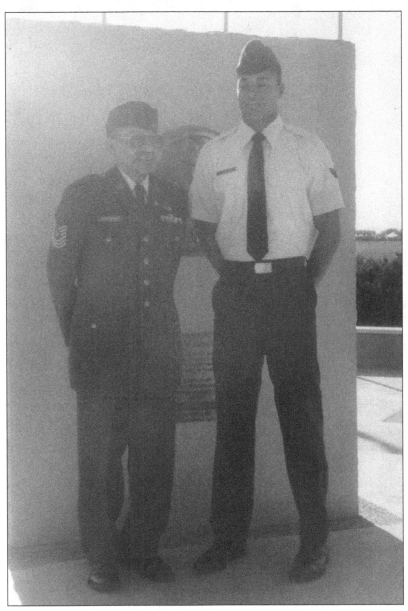

Me and Sgt. Jack at graduation from basic training.

EVOLUTION NO. 5

These are the facts, and they are undisputed. Your problems and your past aren't on anybody else's agenda. Not really. You may have a few people in your inner circle who care about what you're going through, but for the most part, no one cares that much because they're dealing with their own issues and focused on their own lives.

I learned that the hard way. On our drive from Buffalo to 117 South McGuire Street in Brazil, Indiana when I was eight years old, I assumed I was going to walk into the biggest pity party of all time. I expected balloons, cake, ice cream, and big warm hugs. Instead, it was as if all the pain and terror never happened. Sgt. Jack didn't deal in pity. He was out to harden my shell, and that's exactly what he did.

Pity is a soothing balm that turns toxic. At first, when your family and friends commiserate with you and validate the reasons you have for grumbling about your circumstances, it lands like sympathy. But the more comfort pity brings you, the more external validation you'll crave and the less independent you will become. Which will make it that much more difficult for you to gain any traction in life. That's the vicious cycle of pity. It saps self-esteem and inner strength, which makes it harder to succeed, and with each subsequent failure, you will be more tempted to pity yourself.

Look, I get it. Life isn't fair or easy. A lot of us are doing a job that we don't want to do. We feel we are above the tasks coming our way and that the world, or God, or the fates have sentenced us to live in a box we do not belong in. When I was a night-shift security guard at a local hospital, I felt that work was beneath me, so I showed up every night with a voice in my head screaming, *I don't want to be here!* And that infected everything about my life. I ate my feelings, blew up, and slipped into a deep depression. I wanted a different life, but my bad attitude made it impossible to create one.

Every minute you spend feeling sorry for yourself is another minute not getting better, another morning you miss at the gym, another evening wasted without studying. Another day burned when you didn't make any progress toward your dreams, ambitions, and deepest desires. The ones you've had in your head and heart your entire life.

Every minute you spend feeling sorry for yourself is another minute spent in the dungeon thinking about what you lost or the opportunities that have been snatched away or squandered, which inevitably leads to the Great Depression. When you are depressed, you are likely to believe that nobody understands you or your plight. I used to think that way. But when Sgt. Jack banged that trash can lid inches from my ear in the morning, he was telling me I wasn't the only little boy who got whipped or suffered from toxic stress. Sometimes, the emotions we feel are a product of a horrible past. Sometimes, we just don't want to get up at 0500 and do hours of chores before school because it sucks. Sgt. Jack expected me to perform no matter what I'd been through or what time it was.

In response, my feelings got hurt. I stalled getting out of bed until the last possible moment and slouched my way through my mornings as part of a mindless, mopey rebellion. He didn't care. That grass still needed to be cut, the leaves needed to be raked, and the weeds needed to be pulled. No matter how much I belly-ached, this work needed to get done, and it would get done by me. My feelings were costing me a ton of time because no matter how I felt, there was a task in front of me, and that's all that mattered in the present moment.

The only thing that ever matters is the present moment. Yet too many people let their depression or regret hijack their day. They let their feelings about the past hijack their lives. Perhaps their fiancé left them at the altar, or they got fired without cause. Guess what? One day, they will pan back and realize that nobody cared about any of that but them. I don't care what you've been through. I can feel bad for you. I can have sympathy for you, but my sympathy won't get you anywhere. When I was a young, damaged kid, feeling sorry for myself didn't help me. What helped was cleaning those whitewalls right the first time.

We cannot get time back, so we must be minute hoarders. The earlier I get up, the more I do. The less time I stay in pity-party-feel-sorry-for-myself land, the stronger I become and the more daylight I see between me and everyone else. When you separate yourself from the pack by cultivating the values and priorities that lead to greatness, mountains of adversity and hardship become speed bumps, and that makes it easier to adapt to the road ahead and build the new life or sense of self you crave.

When I went to live with Sgt. Jack, I was forced to adapt extremely fast. Everyone was hard on me my whole life, but I came out of all that with lessons learned that stuck with me. Those who learn to adapt survive and thrive. Don't feel sorry for yourself. Get strategic. Attack the problem.

When you adapt, you will begin to see everything that comes your way as a stepping stone on your progression toward a higher plane. High-paying, esteemed jobs are generally not entry level. You have to start somewhere, but most people see the thankless tasks that must be completed in order to advance as burdens instead of opportunities. That makes it impossible for them to learn. You've got to find the lesson in every menial task or low-wage job. That requires humility. I wasn't humble enough to appreciate my experience in security, so my attitude was foul. I thought I deserved much better, oblivious to the fact that almost everybody starts at the bottom and, from there, it's attitude and action that determine the future.

Humility is the antidote to self-pity. It keeps you rooted in reality and your emotions in check. I'm not suggesting you should be satisfied with an entry-level job. I'm never satisfied, but you must appreciate what you have while staying hungry enough to learn everything you can. You need to learn to wash the dishes, flip the burgers, sweat over the deep fryer, sweep up the job site, work in the mailroom, and answer the phones. That's how you build proficiency. It's important to learn every aspect of any business before you move up. You can't rise if you're weighed down by bitterness and entitlement. Humility hardens your spine and encourages you to stand tall, secure in yourself no matter what anyone else thinks. And that has tremendous value.

I once heard a story about a Master Sergeant in the Army named William Crawford that exemplifies the power of humility. He retired in 1967 and took a job as a janitor at the Air Force Academy in Colorado Springs. The cadets he cleaned up after paid him little mind, in part because he was reportedly painfully shy but also because these cadets were elite students on an officer track, and Master Sergeant Crawford was just a janitor. Or so they thought. They had no clue that he was also a war hero.

In September 1943, the 36th Infantry Division was getting blitzed by German machine-gun fire and mortars during a pivotal World War II battle for a piece of Italian real estate known as Hill 424. The Americans were pinned down with no escape route until Crawford spied three machine-gun nests and crawled beneath rivers of bullets to toss a grenade into each of them. His bravery saved lives and allowed his company to advance to safe ground, and after the third direct hit, the Germans abandoned Hill 424, but not before they took Crawford prisoner.

Presumed to be killed in action, tales of his heroism spread among infantrymen and traveled up the chain of command. In 1944, he was awarded the Medal of Honor, the highest decoration in the U.S. military. Because everyone thought he was dead, his father accepted the medal on his behalf. Later that same year, he was found in a liberated POW camp, oblivious to the hype surrounding his name.

In 1976, an Academy cadet and his roommate read about that battle and connected the dots. Their humble janitor had won the Medal of Honor! Can you imagine what went through their heads? The Medal of Honor speaks to everything a military person reveres. Not the medal itself, but the courage and selflessness inside the human being who earned that medal.

Those students wanted to be him, and there he was, mopping their floors and cleaning their bathrooms every day. Master Sergeant Crawford was a walking lesson in self-esteem, courage, character, and, especially, humility.

The way I see it, Master Sergeant William Crawford had figured it out. The Medal of Honor didn't change him. He rose to prominence by staying humble and risking his own life to save others and retired into the service of others. It was never about him, and that gave him strength.

People who feel sorry for themselves are obsessed with their own problems and their own fate. Is that really much different than the greedy and egotistical people who want to feel better than everybody else? The higher I climb in my life, the more I realize how much I need to mop that floor. Because that's where all the knowledge is. There is no grit at the top, no tests of resolve in steak dinners, five-star hotels, or spa treatments. Once you make it in this world, you have to freefall back to the bottom in some way to keep learning and growing.

I call this "trained humility." It's a shedding of your skin that allows you to take on a mission that no one else can see and do whatever needs to be done next. Trained humility is service but also strength. Because, when you are humble enough to remember that you'll never know it all, each lesson you learn only makes you hungrier to learn more, and that will put you on a path that guarantees you will grow all the way to the grave.

> Continued growth only comes when you are willing to be humble. #TrainedHumility #NeverFinished

CHAPTER SIX

THE ART OF GETTING HIT IN THE MOUTH

Leadville reminded me of what I'd been missing in my life for way too long: the steep trails, the waves of pain and exhaustion, and yet another cage match with my own demons. I appreciated having a pacer and being able to share the experience with Kish for the first time. I even relished the aftermath, and I left Colorado wanting more.

The following week, I helped my mom move from Nashville to Las Vegas. On the twenty-six-hour drive, I had plenty of time to complete my After Action Report and review each aspect of the race. One thing about Leadville that I kept coming back to was how much bigger the sport of ultra running had become since my heyday. Back then, 100-milers were run by hard-core endurance athletes like me who sought deeper water. That no longer seemed to be the case. There was great beauty in that. It was evidence that more people were digging deeper. They were curious. They craved more self-knowledge and were willing to pay the toll in pain and suffering. I respected that, but if one hundred miles had become accessible, where was the new deep end?

That thought both excited and unnerved me because it implied that, despite all I'd done in the past, there was still more to give and a lot further to go. I knew that, of course. I preach it all the time, but now I felt it like a slap in the face I didn't see coming.

It's funny how our goals are only as elastic as our sense of self, of who we are and what we think we can accomplish. If all you've ever done is run three miles at a clip, then a ten-mile run can feel as far as the moon. Your mind will compile reasons why that distance is beyond you, and you may believe them. If ten becomes the new normal, then a half or full marathon may be the next step. After a marathon comes ultra. Each time you level up, your mind will step in like an overbearing chaperone and try to shut down the party. That very dynamic was playing out in my own mind on the long drive.

I flashed to a thirty-mile run I'd done with Cameron Hanes in Oregon back in December 2018. While we hammered the trails around his hometown, he gushed about a brand-new race he'd finished two months earlier. It wasn't a 100-miler. It was a 240.3-mile trail race with nearly thirty thousand feet of elevation gain (that's more than the elevation of Mount Everest) among the red-rock formations, sheer drop-offs, and desolated peaks of Moab, Utah. Two hundred and forty miles? Was that the new deep end?

When I was learning to swim as a teenager, I spent all my time in the shallow end of the pool because there was no fear there. Even after I'd become proficient, I swam laps in the shallow end because it soothed me knowing that with each stroke, I almost scraped bottom. If I got too tired or wanted to quit, I could simply stand up, and that gave me both comfort and confidence. It allowed me to work on my stroke without fear getting in the way. There is nothing inherently wrong with that, as long as we are clear that the shallow-end work we put in is all about preparation for the deep end. But that was not my mindset at that point in my life.

The way the pool complex was laid out made it impossible to ignore the deep end. Each day I left the locker room, I had to walk by the ten-foot section. Occasionally, I stepped to the ledge and looked down. That ten-foot floor felt bottomless to me, so I tucked tail and strolled toward the cozy little three-foot marker. With each step, my dread faded while my comfort swelled, and that played with my psyche. I did my best to clear it out of my mind as I swam, but it lodged in there like a thorn, lap after lap, day after day.

When something continually looms in the back of your mind like a taunting, that's an alarm. It's a signal that you need to evaluate and address that issue, or it may become a life-long fear, looming larger each day until it morphs into an obstacle you may never overcome. There is nothing wrong with being afraid or hesitant. We all have our reasons for remaining in the shallow end, but we must make our shallow end a training ground. Too often, we treat our training terrain as a La-Z-Boy. We lay back, get comfy, and then have the audacity to wonder why our lives aren't getting any better while we do the same things we've always done. I should have been using my time in the shallow end as mental preparation, imagining deep water with every stroke.

You have to train your mind as if you are already there. If you get tired while swimming laps in the shallow end, don't give yourself the option of standing up in the middle of the lane. Your only resting point should be the gunnel at the other end of the pool. That way, when you get to the ten-foot end, you know from experience that you can make the distance. But back then, I was merely a survivor. I wasn't a warrior capable of thriving in discomfort, so I chose to bury my dread and logged my pool hours in the shallows with no end in sight.

A lot of us grow out of life's shallow end but stay there because we fear the unknown. I'm thinking of those who remain in a secure job they hate instead of cutting ties and starting up their own business or applying for a new position elsewhere. Most are intimidated by an unknown future filled with variables and consequences they can't control or foresee. I know a person who ran other people's thriving businesses for twenty years but was afraid to run her own. She knew every aspect of what it took to become a successful entrepreneur, but rather than acknowledge her experience and use it as a confidence supply, she let her irrational fears keep her running in place for someone else. You need to evaluate what you are feeling. Not every emotion deserves to be ratified. Remember, if you stay where you've always been, you will never learn if you have what it takes to venture into the deep water.

I felt a glimmer of that old foreboding as we zoomed through the Southwest on the way to Nevada with Moab on my mind. I shook my head in disbelief. Was my mind still trying to stop me after all these years? I thought I'd tamed that monster. And I had, but Moab 240 was something entirely new for me, so fear was a natural response. By then, I knew that there were no tricks around fear. The only way to neutralize it was to commit to doing the thing that freaked me out and then proceed to outsmart my fear through knowledge and preparation.

That night, I googled the race and surveyed the course. It was a roller coaster, traveling up and down from four thousand feet in elevation to 10,500 feet and back again. The weather would be unpredictable, with the potential to deliver serious heat and extreme cold. The distances between aid stations, ranging from nine to nineteen miles, were more than in any other event I had ever done, so I would have to haul a lot more gear than I did for Leadville. The suck factor would be high, but you had 110 hours to finish, which meant you could break it up if you wanted to. A lot of people did, but that's not how I tackle these events. I run straight through and tempt the course to reveal just how fit I am, physically and mentally.

On August 23, I emailed race headquarters in Moab and inquired about signing up. I received a reply within twenty-four hours. The race was scheduled for early October, and I could still apply for a spot. That gave me six weeks to train, and those weeks were already packed with multiple speaking gigs, work commitments, and a lot of travel. All good. I'd find the time to put in the 100-mile weeks required to be ready for the longest run of my career.

Race day was on us in a blink. I gathered with 108 runners from all over the world before dawn on October 11 in Moab, Utah. Some pumped their fists. Others high-fived. They were trying to get motivated to take on hell as if getting happy would insulate them from the reality of what they'd signed up for. That's not me. When I toe the line, I get real quiet. Almost like I'm filing into a funeral. I know the race will bleed the life out of all of us, some more than others, so I grieve for the misery to come. Right up until the horn sounds.

As usual, my leg muscles started out tight. While they were stronger and in better condition than they'd been going into Leadville, my knees were sore. Especially my left knee. During training, it had gotten to the point where I could barely step off a curb without cringing. It took thirty minutes of hobbling before I loosened up enough to find my stride. That became normal. The pain always faded to manageable, and my range of motion tended to kick in once I was warmed up, but I had never run 240 miles in one chunk before. Would my knees last that long?

Moab 240 was a different animal in many ways. It wasn't simply the distance or altitude. The course was a single loop—a network of singletrack trails, sloping rock, open desert, and fire roads—but it wasn't fully marked, so we had to download and mind a particular GPS app on our phones to make sure we stayed on course. Also, we were required to carry a survival kit along with our other gear because there were sections that were inaccessible to our crews or race staff. We had to be able to fend for ourselves and navigate in the wild. This was more than a race. It was a true adventure.

My initial test came right after meeting up with my crew for the first time at mile 17.8, where I stopped long enough to stuff my pack with everything I'd need for the next fifty-five miles. Although there would be aid stations, they were not accessible to crews, which meant I wouldn't see mine again until mile seventy-two. I grabbed gels, powders, extra food and batteries, and a back-up headlamp. I had a 1.5-liter bladder zipped into my pack and two water bottles slotted into the pack's shoulder pockets. But what made the next ten hours so hard wasn't the length or the extra weight. It was the temperature.

The first seventy-two miles of the course ran across a blend of terrain. At times, we were on trails, but without warning, the trail would disappear from under our feet, and I'd find myself running down a sloping rock face wondering where it went. Early on, there was a cluster of ten of us or so out there, our heads on a swivel, checking the app to see if our blinking triangle was still on the dotted line. After four or five hours, we were all strung out, and then, it was just me, out there alone, navigating on the run.

I didn't mind being alone because it kept me thinking, and the complex terrain demanded that I keep my situational awareness (SA) way up. I dialed in my nutrition and hydration, making sure to eat and drink at planned intervals regardless of how good I felt. Any blip in the trail, any potential wrong turn, made me stop and locate where I was and where I needed to be. Sometimes, the cross-country sections lasted a mile or longer. Other times, we were on a distinct trail or road for hours. I was running well, and all was going according to plan until I passed the fifty-mile mark. That's when the desert turned cold. The sun was still up, but the wind was unseasonably crisp, and that was bad news.

I have a condition called Raynaud's phenomenon. In cold weather, the blood flow to my extremities becomes restricted, and blood pools in my core. Back when I was stationed in Chicago and running ultras almost every weekend, I ran during the brutal Chicago winter armed with two layers of thin gloves beneath a pair of ski gloves. Over all of that, I'd pull on thick wool socks, and even then, my hands would be jacked up. I bought a pair of battery-powered, heated gloves just before my Frozen Otter race in 2014, which kept my hands at normal body temperature and enabled my blood to keep flowing. I won that race in part because of those gloves.

I brought those same heated gloves with me to Utah, but Moab in early October wasn't supposed to be anywhere close to as cold as mid-winter in Chicago, and because I had to carry all my own gear and was due to see my crew again at mile 72.3 not long after sunset, I didn't think it made sense to pack the gloves and the bulky batteries. My strategy for races like this has always been to keep everything simple and light. I race streamlined.

I hadn't guessed my fingers would stiffen up from the cold with the sun still out. I knew they might soon become useless, so I stopped, pulled on a pair of thin gloves—which were essentially glove liners—removed my bladder from my pack, and secured it against my chest. I'd had the bladder and drinking hose freeze up in races before—including at Frozen Otter—and I couldn't afford to be dehydrated and freezing at the same time.

There was an aid station at mile 57.3 kitted out with water and food stands—they had someone grilling burgers and another stirring a pot of soup. There was plenty of seating so runners could kick back and eat and drink their fill, but it wasn't a crew meet-up, so the one thing I needed most—my heated gloves—remained out of reach. I didn't eat too much, and though my fingers had lost dexterity, I managed to refill my bladder. After that, there wasn't much to do but keep pushing while the sun slanted lower and lower in the sky.

Thanks to my Raynaud's, my hands and feet felt as heavy and inflexible as ice bricks, my fingers were frozen stiff, but my chest was steaming because so much warm blood had pooled in my torso. That made me thirsty, and I sucked my bladder dry by mile sixty-four. I still had two full water bottles, but I couldn't drink from them because they were the type that I needed to squeeze to get a flow. I brainstormed how to take the lid off with my mouth and could have done it if I'd stopped to take the time, but that would have made me even colder, so I decided against it. I was extremely hungry but couldn't access the food in my pack because my fingers were so wrecked. All I could think about was reaching the aid station to get those heated gloves on my hands.

Alone beneath starry skies, I zeroed in on staying on course and on task. That meant minding the trail and GPS tracker while keeping a steady pace, but time ticks slowly when you're freezing and thirsty and you know you could solve your problems if only your hands worked. I wasn't surprised to feel my energy drain away. My hands hadn't been this cold since SEAL training, and I leaned into those memories to push me uphill. Once again, I called upon past triumphs to push me forward. I wouldn't let myself complain about the fact that my body had begun to betray me yet again. I blocked that out and ran on. Somehow, I made it and slow jogged into the 72.3-mile aid station dehydrated and cold all the way through.

It was hella dark. There were dozens of support crews spread out on flat patches of dirt on both sides of a gravel road in the middle of nowhere. My bones rattled but only for as long as it took to register what was happening and find my team. Then, I reined it in. I didn't want to show my crew so much as a twitch. Crewing races is thankless enough. I didn't need them concerned about anything beyond getting me ready for the next leg.

Kish was the only one who knew about my Raynaud's, and she quickly passed my heated gloves to Jason, one of our crew, who passed them to me. He figured I could put them on myself but watched me peel my thin gloves off my fingers with my teeth and saw that they had become ghost-white. When a Black man's fingers are white as fresh snow, you know something is truly jacked up! He did his best to stuff my frozen hands into the gloves. It was like dressing a baby. He had to force each finger into place, one by one.

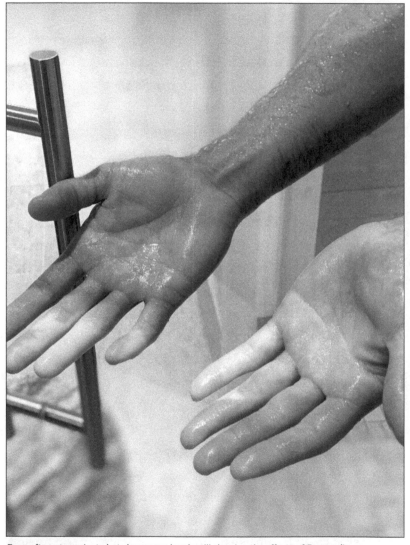

Even after a ten-minute hot shower, my hands still showing the effects of Raynaud's

My hands weren't the only issue. Something was off with my lungs. While I have had respiratory problems in the past when it got cold, this felt different. I filed that concern away and focused on hydration, getting some food in me, and warming up. The heated gloves—which by now were covered by an even thicker pair of larger gloves—thawed my hands out, and I figured as my blood flow shifted back toward normal, my lungs would find some relief. All of that seemed to hold true because within fifteen minutes, I was energized and ready to get back out on the course.

With a pacer by my side, I found a rhythm and started devouring miles as we rolled through Moab's signature red-rock desert countryside under a blizzard of stars. Before long, I was in and out of the next aid station and running with my next pacer along a trail that became a rocky razor's edge. I felt comfortable, but Joe, my pacer for this leg, was freaked out when that trail skirted a deep crater. I peered over the edge. A deep abyss swallowed the glow of my headlamp. The only thing I could see clearly was that now was not the time to lose our footing. We checked into the next aid station at mile 102.3, approximately twenty-one hours into the race and in second place.

That didn't mean a whole lot. I was running well, so far, but we weren't even halfway done. I flashed back to the start, when so many runners were giddy and excited. I wondered how they felt now. Exhausted? Cold? Scared? Were they still as motivated as they were one hundred miles ago? That's why I never get emotional or over-excited at the beginning of something hard. The same is true when it comes to monitoring my progress. I never celebrate anything in the middle of a race. Better to stay calm, focused on my own effort, and aware that what I've gotten myself into is not a game and that there are hungry forces well beyond my control waiting to pounce from behind. A 240-mile run will never be a joy ride. If you're feeling happy with yourself, odds are the tide is about to turn.

That is why it's so important to stay humble and keep that SA up at all times, a lesson I would relearn the hard way as we left the aid station by the light of our headlamps and ran onto a wide gravel road. The sun rose while we ran, and with my new pacer in charge of lead navigation duties and the leader's fresh footprints to follow, I clocked into autopilot. I even put my phone away, the one with the GPS app I'd downloaded for the race. What did I need that for with my co-pilot on nav duty?

There are three crucial requirements to maintaining a high level of SA. The first is astute perception. You need to see the environment clearly. That means knowing where you are on the map and having a good idea where the pitfalls might lie. Sometimes, the pitfall might be a member of your team who isn't as squared away as you'd expected.

It also requires a 360-degree comprehension of the current situation. You must understand the entire picture and take the time to investigate blind spots—areas you might not otherwise see because of exhaustion or low light. You also better have a plan to compensate for any limitations you identify.

Finally, there is projection. Based on your perception and comprehension, what will your future status be? You can't make decisions based solely on the present. You need to think like a chess master and strategize several moves down the line. Unfortunately for me, I screwed that all up.

When we hit an intersection near the bottom of a long descent, my pacer read the footprints and kept on running, and I followed. A few clicks down the road, I noticed that those footprints had turned around but didn't give it a second thought because I trusted my pacer and never checked the GPS to confirm we were still on course. We just kept right on going.

Kish was tracking our progress on her phone using the race leaderboard, which updated our location every five minutes. She could see that I was floating farther and farther out of bounds, and it stressed her out. Race HQ noticed too, and, like Kish, they sent messages and tried to call us for two and a half hours, but my pacer's phone was out of range and mine was packed away. We didn't know that the race leader had made the same wrong turn we did, but his phone somehow had reception, and he answered when headquarters called to alert him. That's why those footprints doubled back after a couple of miles while we kept going for more than ten.

Oct 11	11:25 AM	000.21?	Moab, UT	Incoming, CL
Oct 11	11:47 AM	239.94?	Moab, UT	Bonita Spg, FL
Oct 11	11:53 AM	615.727	Moab, UT	Nashville, TN
Oct 12	5:58 AM	530.42?	Moab, UT	Incoming, CL
Oct 12	6:01 AM	850.87?	Moab, UT	Tallahasse, FL
Oct 12	6:01 AM	000.00?	Moab, UT	Voice Mail, CL
Oct 12	6:01 AM	917.602	Moab, UT	Queens, NY
Oct 12	6:02 AM	850.87?	Moab, UT	Tallahasse, FL
Oct 12	6:02 AM	850.879	Moab, UT	Tallahasse, FL
Oct 12	6:02 AM	917.602	Moab, UT	Queens, NY
Oct 12	6:02 AM	850.879	Moab, UT	Tallahasse, FL
Oct 12	6:06 AM	850.879	Moab, UT	Tallahasse, FL
Oct 12	6:06 AM	530.428	Moab, UT	Loyalton, CA
Oct 12	6:08 AM	850.879	Moab, UT	Tallahasse, FL
Oct 12	6:10 AM	850.879	Moab, UT	Tallahasse, FL
Oct 12	6:11 AM	917.602	Moab, UT	Queens, NY
Oct 12	6:24 AM	850.879	Moab, UT	Tallahasse, FL
Oct 12	6:34 AM	917.602	Moab, UT	Queens, NY

Kish frantically calling because we were off course

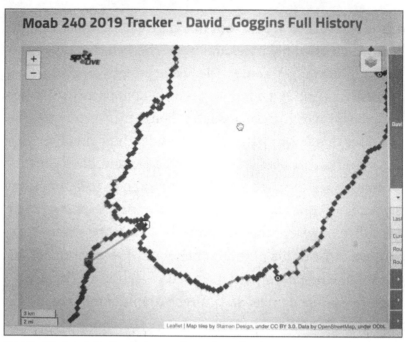

The tail of the loop is the Goggins bonus miles section and each square represents a five minute update.

Part of me sensed we were lost, but I didn't realize that my pacer hadn't downloaded the GPS app properly because I never spot-checked him. Spot checks are a regular part of Ranger School. Each candidate is required to carry several specific items in their bag throughout training, and Ranger Instructors are known to stop and ask random candidates to pull out any one of those specific items at any time. That's a spot check. I should have spot-checked my pacer's phone and made 100 percent sure the app was operational before we left the aid station. Not because I didn't trust him, but because it was four in the morning and neither of us had slept. When I saw the footprints disappear, I missed another opportunity to double-check that we were still on course.

We hadn't seen a marker in miles, and both of us were out

of food and water by the time we reached the next unmarked intersection. That's when his phone blew up with dozens of text messages and missed calls from Kish. He stopped cold, his phone in his hand, with a blank look on his face. He didn't even have to say it. Without a word, I turned and started running back in the other direction.

Was I angry? Not really. Headquarters had been clear that the course was unmarked in many places, which is why I'd paid close attention to my GPS for the first 72.3 miles. But as soon as I picked up my pacers, I left everything up to them, and whenever I go into a non-thinking mode, I always fail. It happened at Delta Selection, and it happened again in Moab. SA is one of my greatest strengths. I take pride in reading terrain, being in tune with myself, and dialing in situations, and whenever my SA drops, whatever I've engaged in falls apart like instant karma.

I had my reasons for handing off nav duty. I was trying to run my race straight through without any sleep. I knew that would take over two and a half days, and I thought it would be more manageable if all I had to do was run and focus on my form, nutrition, and hydration so I could break through any performance barriers and deal with any discomfort that popped up. Remember, I'd already been running for twenty-four hours by the time we made that wrong turn. I was exhausted, and it felt good not to have to think so much. But there is never a time in your life where you should give in to that autopilot mentality.

Before the race, I explained to my pacers that their only job was to not get me lost, which I considered a worst-case scenario. Now that we were here, what good would blowing up at my pacer do? That would have made a bad problem even worse. We needed to focus on getting back on course. Plus, I still needed his help to finish the race. I couldn't shatter his confidence and morale or turn the other crew members against him. Especially since I was the one at fault.

You never want to rely on someone else to lead you in your race. I should have used my pacer as a backstop navigator and kept my eyes on my own GPS the entire time. You cannot miss a turn! And any time you think you may have missed something, you must stop and nuke it right then. I should have had my phone out and checked the GPS app every five to ten minutes if not every mile, but I got lazy because my brain craved a break. I knew 240 miles were no joke and demanded dedication and perseverance, yet I let someone else navigate for me and never even spot-checked them. I could choose to be upset at them if I wanted to, but the only person accountable for this mess was me.

Too many leaders deflect blame and point fingers instead of calling themselves out, but when they do that, nothing gets fixed in the short or long term. I immediately recognized that I allowed the worst-case scenario to happen, and that enabled me to move forward and deal with the ramifications that much faster. Once a mistake has been made in the heat of battle, the only thing that matters is dealing with the aftermath with a clear head. Figuring out where, when, and how things went wrong is important, but all evaluations must wait until the race is over. And now, I was in two races at once: Moab 240, and the race to get to the thyroid medication that awaited me at the next aid station.

When I don't take my thyroid meds, my body goes haywire. When it's really hot, I can feel like I'm freezing. It can also make me slow and sluggish, as if I'm only half-awake, because a malfunctioning thyroid messes with your metabolism. I knew I had drop-dead times for meds, so why hadn't I been carrying them with me? At the last aid station, Kish had them in a baggie ready to go, but I was running really well, and even though I knew I'd be cutting it close, I was confident I would make it to my meds in time given my steady pace. These are the exact mistakes you make when you assume smooth sailing, and the crucible of ultra is built to expose any and all wrong turns and bad choices. This had now become a very bad situation.

After running a total of approximately fifteen miles off course, a race official pulled up in a vehicle a couple miles from our wrong turn. They drove us back to that fateful intersection, which was now clearly marked with signage to spare the runners behind me, but we were still fifteen miles from the next aid station and out of food and water, and I was in dire need of my meds. Headquarters gave Kish permission to meet us on course, but by then, my condition had deteriorated. My core temperature was plummeting, my lungs were heavy, and I knew that if I continued to run, I would become a medical risk.

There were still 135 miles to go in the race, and though I gulped my meds as soon as Kish arrived, my thyroid needed time to reset so my body temperature could normalize. I decided to rest with no idea how long that process might take. I'd already run 120 miles. Predictably, within an hour, my body reacted as if the race was over. I started to swell and tighten up as my muscles shifted into recovery mode.

This would be a problem.

I'd been dealing with my thyroid issue for years. A lot of people in the military, especially those of us in Special Operations, get diagnosed with hypothyroidism because our adrenals are constantly attacked during training and combat—there were forty thousand cases documented between 2008 and 2017. But I'd been living on a fight-or-flight cocktail of hormones ever since I was a young kid. Special Ops just finished the job of burning out my adrenal glands. Once the adrenals shut down, the body attempts to get what it needs by tapping the thyroid. The thyroid is the master computer of the endocrine system, and when it is over-taxed, our metabolism—the process of converting what we drink and eat into energy—becomes impaired, which can cause a cascade of consequences.

Thanks in part to my stretching regimen, my adrenals had recovered enough in recent years to stop attacking the thyroid, which allowed it to begin healing. In fact, it turned out that my AFib episode over Christmas was sparked by a heavier-than-necessary dose of thyroid medication. Since then, my doctors and I had been experimenting with lower dosages. I've been a sickly boy all my life. If my body were only healthy and whole, there would be no telling what I might be able to accomplish.

In the end, I was down for twelve hours, and while that amount of rest might sound like it could help me later in the race, it is actually quite the opposite. By the time I was back on the trail, my legs felt like they were made out of stone. I was that stiff and swollen. And I had fallen from second to something like eightieth place, which was more or less dead last. I had every excuse to quit—my luck had soured, my health was compromised, and I'd lost my SA at a crucial time. My race was completely hijacked, and I had over half the distance still to go! Some might look at that version of events and think all was lost, but I knew from experience that the best life lessons don't appear when things go well. It's when all your goals and pretty plans burn to ash that you can see your flaws and learn more about yourself.

You must take advantage of any opportunity to strengthen your resolve because when life hits you in the mouth, you will need that resolve. Of course, knowing that doesn't make it easy to reengage when everything goes sideways. Actually getting out there and running the last 135 miles demanded a level of focus and commitment that is hard to find when you've been down and out for half a day. Fortunately, I'd been in similar situations so many times before. I knew what to do.

For starters, I had to stay locked in mentally. A lot of people fall down when they get smacked, and when they hit the ground, they lose all momentum. Not just physically but mentally because they are humiliated, and when you are humiliated, it is impossible to make any sort of progress. We must learn how to absorb life's haymakers without getting knocked down. Because picking yourself up off the canvas is the hardest, longest step of all as you fight to regain your momentum. Yes, I had to shut it down for half a day. Yes, all the goals I had for Moab 240 had been obliterated. Yes, my body was a mess, but mentally, I was still on my feet and in the race because I'm not living life for the same reasons as almost everyone else.

The rewards I seek are internal, and if you have that mindset, you will find opportunities for growth everywhere. During tough times, that growth can be exponential. I wasn't going to win the race or finish in a respectable time, but I had been gifted another rare opportunity to test myself in adverse conditions and become more. If anything, my desire to finish had only grown thanks to the mess I'd made.

At the same time, I needed to ease some of the pressure I'd placed on myself. Pressure comes with high expectations, which is great because it can bring out your best, but there are times when it can be more helpful to offload pressure. When you are exhausted, it is vital to remain in control of your thoughts and emotions so you can make decisions with your right mind. Choosing to relieve pressure allows you to do that.

When the pressure is high, you develop blinders that limit perspective. That's great for certain situations that demand a hyper focus, but when you're engaged in something that demands your maximum endurance, it's better to broaden your perspective and your awareness to absorb more of the experience, which enables maximum growth both during the event and in the days and weeks to follow. Besides, if you allow that unrelenting pressure to build, you're liable to snap and make a bad situation a whole lot worse. Remember, the goal is always to complete the mission—whatever it may be—with no regrets and a clear head, so you can use it to progress in life.

Cultivating a willingness to succeed despite any and all circumstances is the most important variable of the reengagement equation. Your willingness to succeed builds self-esteem. It broadens your concept of your own capability, yet it is the first thing we lose touch with when things go bad. After that, giving up often feels like the sanest option, and maybe it is, but know that quitting chips away at your self-worth and always requires some level of mental rehab. Even if what forces you to quit is an injury or something else beyond your control, you will still have to bounce back from the experience mentally. A successful mission seldom requires any emotional maintenance.

In order to execute on your willingness to succeed, you will need to be able to perform without purpose. You've heard of purpose, that magical missing ingredient crucial to landing a fulfilling career and building a happy life. What if I told you the importance of finding your purpose was overblown? What if there never was any such thing as your good friend purpose? What if it doesn't matter what you do with your time here? What if it's all arbitrary and life doesn't care if you want to be happy? What then?

All I know is this: I am David Goggins. I exist; therefore, I complete what I start. I take pride in my effort and in my performance in all phases of life. Just because I am here! If I'm lost, I will find myself. As long as I'm on planet Earth, I will not half-ass it. Anywhere I lack, I will improve because I exist and I am willing.

This is the mentality we should all strive for when we're stuck. Because when you're in the hurt locker, you must be your own motivator, your own drill instructor. In the dark moments, you must remind yourself why you chose to be there in the first place. That takes an edgy tone. When you're all jacked up and looking for more, the only tone you should allow inside your head is the tone of a warrior. The tone of someone prepared to plunge deep inside their own soul to find the energy they need to keep up the fight and prevail!

In Moab, my willingness to succeed was fueled by my future. I knew the race I had planned to run was over, but as of that moment, next year's race had already begun. My new mission was to sketch out the ultimate blueprint for this course. I'd released the pressure valve, and my entire team was refreshed and ready to scout details with me. Like future bank robbers, masters of disguise returning to the branch day after day to absorb the layout, document the rhythms of the staff, and come up with an unbeatable plan of attack, we would catalog firsthand knowledge of the next 135 miles so in 2020, I would be prepared to blow it up.

Once I started again, I walked for the first ten minutes. My gait was way off. So were my lungs, but when I saw my first headlamp, I felt a little spark. After that, I began to add the pressure back, bit by bit. My pace increased, and my competitive edge resurfaced. I managed to pass two dozen people before hitting the aid station at mile 140.

Kish was next up as pacer, and she had a ball. We'd been running together for years, but this was the first time she was able to check me on a long stretch, and she made it look way too easy. To be fair, the terrain was flat and smooth, but she hadn't slept either. She'd been the crew chief the whole time yet ran like she'd had a full night's sleep. I'd run 157 total miles by then (counting the off-course mileage) and was deep in the hurt locker, while she was checking her phone, collecting footage, and keeping tabs on the crew. Whenever I stopped to walk, she always ran a bit farther ahead to wait for me. She wasn't trying to get under my skin, but I took it as a challenge and was able to pick up my pace enough to pass several dozen runners. Some were walking, others were asleep on the trail or at the aid stations, content to take their time, knowing they had three more days to complete the course. The one person I couldn't keep pace with was Kish, and that's all I cared about! By the time we got to the Rd 46 aid station at mile 167, I was back in the top ten.

But it wasn't time for high-fiving because my lung issues were still there. It didn't matter if I was running or walking, standing up or sitting down, I could not get a full breath. I was freezing too, which was a sign that my thyroid may not have had enough time to completely reset. I felt horrible, but I had weathered a thyroid problem and run through the night for the second night in a row. Pain and discomfort were to be expected.

This aid station had more food stands, and I ate my fill. As I left—a few minutes ahead of my pacer, who was still organizing gear and wasn't ready to go—I wondered if I'd eaten too much because my chest felt very tight. Did I have a digestive issue? I couldn't say for sure, so I continued to troubleshoot. I had a fully loaded pack on my back that was heavy enough to make the chest strap extremely tight. Maybe that was what prevented my lungs from fully expanding? I loosened the strap and felt even worse.

While I had gone farther than this once before, that was back in 2007 and on a flat one-mile track. I had never gone this far on this type of terrain and in these conditions, but I had pushed myself to the limit plenty of times and never felt anything like this. Could it be a sickle cell crisis? If it was, I'd never had one this serious. I couldn't pinpoint the problem, but by the time my pacer caught me, I felt something was extremely wrong.

I told him everything, and as I listened to myself spill my sad story, I couldn't help thinking about all the whiners I'd come across over the years who gave every excuse in the world as to why they couldn't finish whatever it was they'd started. The vast majority of them were simply looking for a way out that allowed them to keep their heads up—like me when I quit Pararescue. I took mental note of all of those people, remembered the scenarios they were in, and kept them on lock in my brain. And here I was sounding just like them.

Whether it is a seven-mile run or a 240-mile run, we all know what it's like to bargain with ourselves to avoid having to do the very thing we said we would. We say we're overworked, overwhelmed, or just over it entirely. I never give in to that because I know there are a lot of people out there who do not have that choice to make. They cannot run at all and wish more than anything that they could.

At the same time, I knew I wasn't merely uncomfortable. I was seriously screwed up! But running Moab 240 had been my choice. Staying in the race had been my choice, and it was a blessing that I had those choices to make. So, like always, I soldiered on. And as the trail wound through farmland and pitched toward the sky and into those mountains that had looked painted against the distant horizon all day, I reminded myself why I wanted to be there. It was for that one second of glory—the biggest high of all time that strikes and fades like a bolt of lightning, but only if you manage to figure out a way to swim through all the pain, overcome every last obstacle, and cross the finish line.

Over the next thirteen miles, we gained 3,500 feet of elevation, and my pace slowed dramatically. Part of that was the incline, but there were times when the footing was bad too. In sections, the trail was covered with slate, shattered cobbles, and boulders. It was really unstable, so I took my time. And after ten miles, I actually started to feel a little better. I didn't feel great, but my condition had improved, and my pacer, who had done due diligence on past performances to gauge how hard I should push on each section, said we were covering this leg at a fast clip. That gave me hope as the trail wound into the alpine forest at just under nine thousand feet and into the Pole Canyon aid station at dusk, where a volunteer griddled fluffy pancakes and handed them out to all comers. My crew was there waiting on me with a syrupy stack and a race update. I had moved all the way up to eighth place.

Even if my problems were digestive, and I wasn't entirely convinced of that, I still had to fuel up. I took the plate from Kish and continued to troubleshoot while I ate. I asked if she had accidentally mixed the wrong powder—something with caffeine—in my water bottles. I have a caffeine intolerance, but Kish knew that and assured me that did not happen. One thing I still hadn't considered was altitude because while we were climbing at times, we were not very high for very long. My lungs had been fine during Leadville just six weeks earlier, and I ran the majority of those one hundred miles above ten thousand feet. The source of my problem remained elusive, and that bothered me because the race was nowhere near done. Anything could happen out there, and sure enough, not long after I made my way out of the aid station, my breathing problems returned.

Within five minutes, I stopped and asked Dan, my pacer for this section, to call Kish and tell her and the crew to stay at Pole Canyon in case we needed to turn around. But I also wanted to give myself every chance to walk through the fire. Maybe it was the pancakes? Last time, I felt better after a couple of hours, and if I could stay upright and on the trail, then it followed that these symptoms might pass again.

Incremental progress is still progress, I said to myself. *One step is all that is required to take the next one.*

With that in mind, I told Dan to call Jennifer again and say we were going to press on and we would let her know if anything changed. We continued climbing into the night toward the highest point in the entire race at 10,500 feet. The protocol was this: take a few steps, double over, and lean heavily on my poles until I could get the few deep breaths necessary to power me forward for another three to five steps, repeat. I couldn't breathe at all while I was moving. It was all panting and gasping. Whenever I stopped to breathe, I could see Dan waiting for me with a concerned look on his face.

"I'm sorry," I gasped. "I'm sorry." I must have said sorry close to three hundred times. I don't know why I kept apologizing. Mostly he responded, "It's not that far to the top." Which was quite comical because I knew we weren't even close! He was trying to spoon-feed me some hope, but hope would not get me to the top. *Nice try, Dan!* I thought to myself.

In the fourth hour, about six miles into the 16.5-mile section—that's right, we were moving at a snail's pace of just over thirty minutes per mile—I finally and abruptly stopped. "This ain't...good," I said, gasping. I was proud of myself for trying, but I still wasn't feeling any better. In fact, my lungs had gotten much worse, and Dan agreed that we should get off the course and find a medic. He dialed Kish and broke the news, and I watched his face fall at her response.

"Hey, man," he said after he hung up. I was still bent over at the waist, begging for oxygen. "I hate to tell you this, but we gotta walk out of here."

He explained that there were only two options. Option one was to descend six miles, back to Pole Canyon. Option two was to keep climbing for nine more miles toward a trailhead where my crew could meet us. None of this came as a surprise to me, as we were on a narrow singletrack. I had been looking for different trails that might offer a possible way out all night but hadn't seen one. The only trail I saw was the one I was walking on, and I knew there was no way a vehicle, an ATV, or anything of the sort could reach me here in no man's land. I also knew for certain there was no helicopter to fly me out of there. The only way out was under my own power.

Going back to Pole Canyon was not an option because despite my wretched condition, I did not intend to quit the race. Somehow, I was still willing—so instead of losing mileage, I opted to continue climbing. This was no longer a race. This had become war, and I was wounded but maintained hope that eventually the medic would dial me in, and I could carry on with the fight.

The night closed in around us as we picked away at the distance. In some spots, the trail was just wide enough to place my feet down one in front of the other. Drop-offs materialized from the shadows without warning. Breathing continued to be a struggle, and I couldn't stop thinking about John Skop, the young, six-foot-two, 225-pound stud who died of pulmonary edema during my third Hell Week.

I would shuffle my feet forward, lean over my poles, close my eyes, and there he was, feverish and jackhammering, suffering from pneumonia and the late stages of pulmonary edema on the pool deck. His skin was almost translucent, his eyes vacant, his breath shallow, just like mine. He looked fragile as porcelain but had no intention of quitting. When he rejoined the caterpillar swim, he was weak because he could barely breathe, and within a few minutes, he was found on the bottom of the pool and could not be resuscitated.

Skop had been trying to become a SEAL at all costs, and I will always respect him for that. I would have done the same thing. There are certain things in life that warrant an "even if I die" mindset. Sometimes, that's a place you have to go, but what's on the other side of that mountain has to be something you want more than anything in the world. However willing I may have been, finishing Moab 240 did not qualify. I'd accomplished enough that finishing the race wouldn't change a thing when it came to how I felt about myself, and I certainly didn't need to die for it.

By then, I suspected I had high-altitude pulmonary edema (HAPE), a dangerous condition in which the lungs fill with blood and plasma. It's a version of what happened to Skop, and it can happen to anybody in the high country, even experienced mountaineers, at relatively low altitudes. I was at close to ten thousand feet, which is not all that high, but because I'd already run over two hundred miles, I was susceptible to anything and everything.

With less than three miles to go before I would reach the top of the peak and the next aid station at mile 201.4, a medic and two members of my crew found us on the trail. Unfortunately, there was nothing the medic could do for me. My choices were to either continue walking all the way to the aid station or stop at a trailhead on the way, where our vehicle was waiting. I knew that after the next aid station, there was a long descent, and despite how bad I felt, I did wonder if my body might be able to bounce back. Then I caught myself.

I'm often mistaken for a masochist. Some people think I push past pain and take unreasonable risks for sport or spectacle, but that's not true. I push a lot harder than most, but I don't do it to injure myself or impress others, and I sure don't want to die. I do it because the body and mind never fail to amaze me. I had no business hiking 16.5 miles in my condition. The last nine felt impossible because I thought I'd reached my physical limit, but when I looked for it, I found more. Whenever I've been challenged, whenever I've been forced to scrap for additional resources to stay afloat, there has always been more. That's why I ride that line: because those dark moments are rare, raw, and beautiful. However, that night, I felt worse than ever, and I knew that any extra stress on my body might be my breaking point. When we reached the trailhead, I left the course to seek medical treatment, which meant, according to the rules, that I was automatically DNF'd.

On the drive to the local hospital, we lost nearly six thousand feet in altitude, and I began hocking up knots of brown phlegm. In the emergency room, the doctor took a chest X-ray that confirmed my air sacs were full of fluid. I had HAPE alright. She checked my vitals, drew blood, gave me a small-volume nebulizer oxygen treatment to open up the lungs, and tested my phlegm to see what kind of infection was present. A few hours later, at around six in the morning, the hospital discharged me with an inhaler that would help keep my lungs opened up.

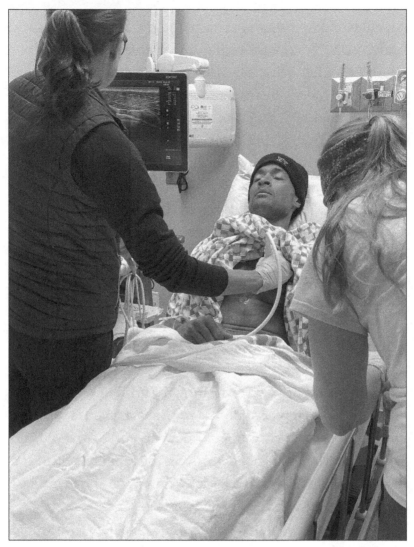

HAPE diagnosis

When Kish and I got back to the condo we'd rented, the rest of our crew was busy packing, cleaning, and getting ready to travel home. The mood was subdued. This race had been tough on everyone. My crew had fought through multiple setbacks and weathered a ton of highs and lows, and while I was proud of running 215 miles with a broken body and considered those last

16.5 miles of slow marching some of the grittiest I'd ever clocked, taking a DNF is a crappy feeling, and everybody knew it.

At least I felt better. By afternoon, I'd stopped coughing up phlegm, and my body temperature and energy levels were back to normal, which told me that my thyroid was functioning again. When I had to take DNFs in the past, there was no quick bounce back. I was down for weeks. This situation was new, and it sent my mind reeling.

There are a lot of people who stay down way too long. They may have been sick as hell but are on the mend, yet when asked how they are feeling, they act like they are no better. In fact, they play it up for pity points. I am not one of those people. The second I feel I can get after it, I am going to get after it. Bottom line: I was struggling with the fact that I was feeling well enough to compete and was in a condo instead of on the trail.

A voice in my head woke me from my fitful slumber at three in the morning. It repeated the same savage mantra over and over. *You're not done yet, Goggins!* I popped up, bleary-eyed and half asleep. There was nobody else in the room but Kish, and she was dead to the world. I lay back down and closed my eyes, but the voice returned. *You are not done yet!*

I knew what I had to do but had no clue how Kish would take it. We'd packed it in. Two members of the crew had already left, and the other two were leaving on flights in a matter of hours, but I would finish the job alone if necessary. I turned and placed my hand on Kish's shoulder. She blinked twice.

"What time does the finish line close?" I asked. Her eyes grew wide. She looked disoriented, so I asked again, "What time does the finish line close?"

Kish knew that what I really wanted to know was if there

was enough time left for me to run the last forty or so miles. The race had started four days ago, but runners had 110 hours to complete it. She sat up and grabbed her phone from the nightstand. "We have fifteen hours," she said.

There was something matter of fact about the way she said it that fed my fire. She may not have understood why I was still holding on to this race, but her mind was made up. She was in, and that's all that mattered. We got up. I rousted the two members of my crew who were still with us and asked if they would be willing to postpone their flights for one more day.

Within a few minutes, we were all in the kitchen arranging our gear and grabbing a quick bite. The little bit of rest had done me good, and while Moab was only at four thousand feet in elevation and things might change when we returned to altitude, I wouldn't be in the high country for long. There was only a mile and a half of climbing, then a long descent back to town. But don't mistake my willingness to finish the job as excitement to get back out there and run another forty miles. I had already run 215 miles over the last four days, and though I felt well enough to get after it, my body had started to recover, which meant I was stiff and very swollen. I knew this would hurt.

Before we left, Kish placed a call to my doctor back home to make sure I wasn't taking any unnecessary risks. After a moment of silence to consider who she was talking to and peruse my thick medical file in her mind, she okayed it. "If you start to feel any symptoms, please stop immediately, leave the course, and return to lower elevation," she said.

On the drive up the mountain, my ears popped, which was a reminder of how much altitude we were gaining. I had no clue what would happen at 10,500 feet, but while I didn't really want to run again, I suspected I was capable, which meant I had to try to finish the job. Completing the blueprint is what excited me, so that's what I focused on.

Kish pulled into the trailhead parking lot near mile marker two hundred, where I had left the course. I was looking to waste no time at altitude. My pacer and I grabbed our gear and headed up the mountain quickly. My team maintained contact for those first two miles to make sure I was okay. My legs were stiff as rocks, and I walked with an unsteady gait, but my breathing was fine. Still, I felt weak and unconfident. This course had gotten the better of me since mile seventy-two, and part of me thought I was either insane or stupid for trying to finish. Probably both.

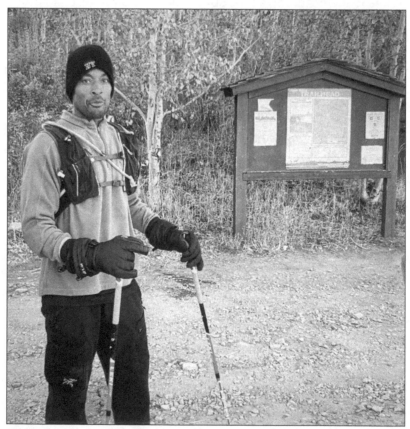

Back at the scene of the crime, mile two hundred

Kish trailed us on the gravel road heading to the mountaintop, and with "Going the Distance" blasting through the open windows, she pulled up alongside and smiled. That anthem was an old friend. We'd shared countless dark times, and it never failed to drown out all my internal chatter and wake up my inner savage. I let the music soak in and found my determination to mark a course that had been kicking my butt for four days.

"I'm back!" I yelled, picking up my pace. "You thought you had me! You thought you had me down! Only for a second. I'm back!"

From then on, it was all growth. The next forty miles were my strongest of the entire race. I hit a level of awareness that allowed me to run free and unpack and examine the previous two hundred-plus miles at the same time. With my feet still on the same ground where I'd come up short, eyes on the rocks and trees that played tricks on me, and my mind on where I screwed up, I was able to complete my ultimate blueprint.

And the most important thing I learned as I descended toward the red rocks of Moab was that 240 miles is an entirely new realm, and my failure came down to a fundamental flaw in my approach. I'd perfected the 100-mile distance. I knew the gear I needed and how to manage the distance with my mind, but that proved irrelevant in Moab. Hundred-milers have aid stations sprinkled every six to ten miles. In Moab, the aid stations were often several hours apart. All but one of the dozens of 100-mile races I'd run were on well-marked courses, so there was no need to prioritize navigation. I'd rocked up like this was just another race, but it was a whole different arena, and that single error led to a cascade of small mistakes that were magnified by the distance into a catastrophe.

Next year, the Moab 240 would be part race, part military

mission. I would imagine the worst-case scenario and work backwards from there so no matter what happened, I would be armed with a plan to remain competitive. I realized that the farther the distance, the more I had to have all the details dialed. There would be no room to take chances with gear or meds. I had to carry it all with me. I couldn't count on bridging great distances between meet-ups with my crew in a timely fashion. I needed to spot-check my pacers, update my phone, and have back-up comms on hand. Normally, I enjoy being unreachable and off grid when I'm trail running, but next year, I would make an exception because that's what the course demands. I worked over dozens of small adjustments in my mind as I flew downhill, my lungs in fine shape, my stride efficient and powerful.

And I reminded myself that in each and every evolution of life, you never want to be the principal reason for a failed mission. Nobody wants to wake up after the race is over wishing they'd been better prepared. If something surprises you in anything you are trying to accomplish these days, with so much free knowledge at our fingertips, it is because you didn't prepare well enough, and there is no excuse for that. Missions may fail for dozens of reasons, which is fine. Make sure it was something beyond your control—an act of God or Mother Nature—that prevented you from achieving your goal. Then, draw up your ultimate blueprint, and try again.

As I ran from a bike trail onto the Moab city streets, I knew I'd make the cut off, but because I'd DNF'd, I didn't have the right to cross the official finish line. For me, that would have to wait until next year. We found a worthy alternative: a random telephone pole, one of several on a busy highway.

As traffic zoomed by, I jogged along the shoulder until my total mileage clicked over to 255—that included the official

240 plus those fifteen unofficial miles. I didn't raise my arms or pump my fists, and nobody seemed to notice one man finish what he started, but I felt a deep sense of satisfaction. There was no fanfare, but there was glory, and it was all inside.

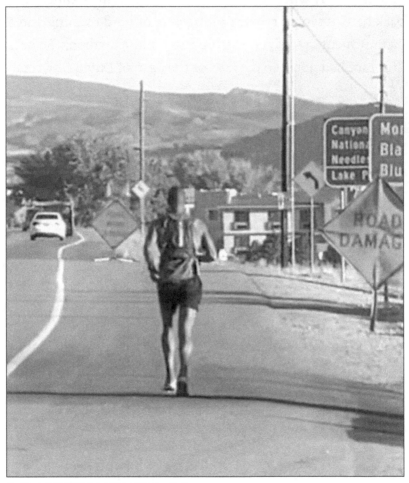

My Moab 240 2019 finish line. All internal glory.

From the outside looking in, my Moab 240 was a disaster. I got lost, nearly froze my tail off, and had multiple medical meltdowns. I went off course twice. It was messy, but I consider it one of my top five performances ever because I never should have completed that distance in the time allowed. But I did. Yes, the scoreboard still read: Moab 1, Goggins 0, but I left Utah with a precious gift.

Unlike during 2018, when I was uncertain about so much, I knew exactly where I would be in twelve months' time: right back here. It would require a long year of hard training and a commitment to studying my blueprint like a textbook. So be it. This race had not seen the last, or the best, of David Goggins!

EVOLUTION NO. 6

S mall minds and weak people kill big dreams. You might have clear goals and be working on yourself every day, but if you have the wrong folks around you, there's a good chance they could be sucking the life right out of you and making sure that you go nowhere.

When I select my crew, I'm not looking for elite runners to pace me. I look for individuals with a foxhole mentality. Of the four men who joined Kish and me in Moab, only one had ever done an ultra before, and two others barely ran twenty miles a week, but I didn't choose them for their running ability; they all understood me. They appreciated my mindset, knew how far I was willing to go, and were ready to do whatever it took to get me there. My success in this race was their only priority. When I told them I was heading back out to finish the job, nobody was surprised. They had been with me all day, knew I was feeling better, and, most importantly, know who I am. They expected me to try and finish. When I knocked on their doors at four in the morning, they were nearly packed for the trail already, with a look on their faces that said, "What took you so long?"

In military speak, the foxhole is a fighting position. In life, it's your inner circle. These are the people you surround yourself with. They know your history and are aware of your future goals and past limitations. But because it's a fighting position, a foxhole can just as easily become your grave. Therefore, it is crucial that you be careful about who you invite in. Whether you are at war, competing in a game, or striving in life, you never want someone in your foxhole who lacks faith or will try to steer you away from your full potential by giving you permission to pack it in or wave the white flag when the situation looks bleak.

You want the husband or wife who, when you snooze that alarm on a freezing mid-winter morning before dawn, shakes you awake so you don't miss your training run. When you're dieting and whine about being bored of eating the same bland foods every day, they remind you of all the progress you have made, of all the hard work you have put in, and happily eat the same bland foods alongside you. When you say you're tired from all the late-night studying, they stay up late with you to help you study.

You want the type of race crew who, when you're suffering on the trail, are inspired by bearing witness to your struggle. They know it is proof of your effort. In turn, their refusal to give up on you can only inspire you to tap the reserves you'd forgotten were there and give more. They know the only time to shut down and walk away is after all options have been exhausted. Even if that means yet another sleepless night or a last-minute change of schedule. When those are the people in your foxhole, how can you not stay in the fight?

Most people don't have a selection process for their foxhole.

They invite all the old cronies and close relatives in by default. As if growing up with someone is the top qualification for fox-hole membership. Old friends are great and shared history is to be respected, but not every person who has been in your life a long time is looking out for your best interests. Some of them are threatened by your growth because of how it impacts them. Some are looking for a friend to keep them company in their unfulfilling lives.

In order to populate your foxhole with the right people, you must first know who you are as an individual. That means shaking off old belief systems—creaky concepts of the world and your place in it—that no longer serve you and the habits and lifestyle that you've outgrown. Any ideas or interests that were impressed upon you by others, whether they be your family, peers, or culture, must be examined consciously so you can see through all of them and discover your own unique individuality. For most people, this is a slow, organic process that can take years, if it happens at all, but if you bring intentionality to it, individuation can be accelerated. Once you find out who you are, the world will start delivering you care packages filled with opportunities that will fuel your quest.

In addition to power eating and spraying cockroaches, I did a lot of searching after I left the Air Force at twenty-four years old. I was looking for my place in the world and tried on different personas and subcultures. I explored becoming a wrestler. I got into powerlifting and thought about competing in that sport, but those weren't honest choices. I didn't burn with a desire to wrestle or lift heavy on stage. All I knew was that I didn't want to be David Goggins anymore. I wanted to be the hardest person ever to live. The problem was I didn't know what that looked like.

It was terrifying to admit that to anyone, including myself, because at the time, I was out of shape, working a low-wage job, and living well beyond my means. How do you go from that to being hard as hell? I had no clue and wondered if I was delusional. Who gave me the right to have such an audacious dream? Even I thought I sounded ridiculous. But as absurd as it may have seemed, I didn't let go of that dream. I let it linger in the back of my brain. Then one day, a care package arrived in the form of a Navy SEAL documentary. And there it was. I finally found a place to start that might just lead me there. My dream no longer felt delusional. It felt possible.

My evolution had begun, but as my Navy SEAL future crystallized over the next several months, I learned that when you change, not everyone in your life will be on board. You will get some serious resistance, and it will be a pain. Everywhere I turned, I found family members, friends, and coworkers resistant to my evolution because they loved the Ecolab-spraying, chocolate-shake-slurping fat boy. At three hundred pounds, I made them feel much better about themselves, which is another way of saying, they were holding me back.

Years later, I learned how common that kind of thing is. Most of the men I recruited into the SEALs confided that their wives, girlfriends, or parents were dead set against something they wanted more than anything in the world. That can be extremely stressful. When you are striving to be you—especially when it involves pushing your limits of pain and suffering or sacrificing life and limb—you do not need to deal with trying to make everybody happy at the same time. When you are conflicted like that, your internal dialogue becomes counterproductive, and when those moments of truth arrive and the quitting mind gets loud, that inner conflict might be the very thing that convinces you to give up.

When I first made the decision to try to become a Navy SEAL, the only person in my foxhole was my mom. She knew what it entailed and was immediately on board. I didn't see any fear in her eyes. While she was worried about me, she believed in what I was doing even more, and that allowed me to train and fight with a clear head and maximum focus. Years later, when I ran Badwater, she was in my crew. I walked one hundred of those 135 miles, and when horseflies were all over me and I was suffering in the heat, she got out of the support vehicle, sobbing. Not because I was in pain, but because she was proud of me. Because I was pushing through it all like a warrior.

Not all friends and loved ones react that way when you change and become committed to perpetual growth. Some are genuinely offended, and you don't need or want their voices in your head. Which is a nice way of saying you may be required to leave some people behind along the way. Who you hang around and speak to on the daily matters. That's why it is not a successful formula for people in drug and alcohol recovery to continue to hang out with the people they used to party with if they want to stay sober. When you evolve, your inner circle must evolve with you. Otherwise, you may subconsciously halt your own growth to avoid outpacing and losing contact with the people who mean a lot to you but may not be able to hang with you.

When there is no one around you who believes in or understands your quest, you must turn your foxhole into a one-man fighting position. That's okay. It is always better to fight alone until you can find people strong enough to fight the good fight with you. There is no time to waste trying to pull deadweight up a hill. I've been there many times, and you must hold out until reinforcements arrive, even if it takes years. Loneliness can be difficult and depleting, but I'd much rather you stay lonely than crawl out of your foxhole and trek back through known territory into the arms of the very people who loved the old you and were never comfortable with your transformation.

Does this mean you have to end all relationships or burn all bridges? No, not necessarily. But doubters must be kept at arm's length, and anyone in your inner circle must accept you for who you are and who you want to become. This may require an adjustment period, and that is understandable. But within a reasonable amount of time, the men and women in your foxhole must, in their words and actions, give you permission to be you.

In 2018, right before I received my VFW award, I realized how much I couldn't stand being retired. I spent hours calling old friends and new contacts in the military, looking for a way back in. I considered reenlisting in Pararescue, but remembering how much I loved Ranger School and Delta Selection, I thought the Army might be a better fit, so I dropped word that I was interested in enlisting as a forty-four-year-old grunt. It didn't take long for a recruiter to reach out. He was convinced he could make it happen, but it meant moving to some backwoods Army base for training.

Kish was not thrilled. She'd worked hard in the corporate world for twenty years, and she did not expect to be living on or around an Army base at that point in her life. She certainly didn't expect me to turn down dozens of lucrative speaking gigs to prepare for a third stint in the military. By then, I was already earning more money for an hour or two of public speaking than I'd earn in a year as a grunt.

I found myself walking on eggshells, wondering if the woman I loved would want to stay with me. At the same time, I knew living someone else's idea of my life is a recipe for misery.

In the end, for a number of reasons, I didn't reenlist. I got into wildland firefighting instead. My mission hadn't changed. I was, and still am, trying to become the hardest person to ever live. That's not an ego trip. It's a way of life. It may be far-fetched and even unachievable, but I remain in service of that vision.

Fast forward a few years, and Kish is most definitely foxhole qualified. Now, she is the one who blocks off the fire season entirely and turns down every speaking inquiry that comes in for those months without even asking me because she understands exactly who I am and what I am about. She knows what my priorities are and fully supports them without question. She admires that I am fulfilled by doing things that most people shy away from and that the lure of money and fame do absolutely nothing for me but leave me feeling empty. She wants me to find my very best.

I'm wired the same way. When Kish confided in me that she wanted to run a sub-3:25 marathon, I helped her train and strategize, and she accomplished her goal with a time of 3:21 in Philadelphia. When she mentioned possibly applying to law school, she received a package of LSAT books at the door the very next day.

Don't ever tell me you want to run a marathon because I will sign you up for a race, monitor your daily training, and run with you. If you tell me you want to be a doctor, I'll be the one who enrolls you in med school while you're sleeping, and you'll wake up to a class first thing in the morning. Most people can't handle that level of intensity. But that's the kind of backing I want. The type that comes with an expectation of effort and demands hours, weeks, and even years of hard work. Because that is exactly what it takes to fulfill lofty ambitions and, more important than that, find out what you are truly capable of.

> Who's in your foxhole? Tag them and tell them why! #Foxhole-
> Mentality #NeverFinished

CHAPTER SEVEN

THE RECKONING

The minute I got home from Moab, I went for a run. Training for next year's race was underway that quickly, and I was fired up! Running had long ago become like breathing to me. It wasn't a hobby; it was almost a subconscious biological reflex. I had to do it. I didn't necessarily enjoy it, but I could tell on that initial eight-mile shakeout that there was going to be something very different about this training block. I could already feel the fire. Day after day, I could not wait to get after it, and I trained with reckless abandon.

My mind was tracking like never before. This wasn't merely about checking some box, this was straight-up redemption. The fitness I gained would also benefit the only other significant event on my 2020 radar, the wildland firefighting season in Montana.

But in April 2020, a few short weeks before I was due to report to work in Missoula, my left knee swelled up like a water balloon. My knees had troubled me periodically since Navy SEAL training, and I wasn't overly concerned at first. I'd been going hard and figured it was due to overuse rather than injury. I ignored the tenderness and ran through the pain for days. My body has been compensating for illness and injury for so long that I figured it was only a matter of time before my quadriceps stabilized my knee joint and the pain faded into the background. But it got worse.

Reluctantly, I traded in the majority of my road miles for a few daily hours on the elliptical trainer. However, firefighting demands a special variety of real-world fitness. To prepare for the infamous 110-pound rucks that awaited me in Montana, I hiked the local trails with a one-hundred-pound pack strapped to my back a couple times a week. It was too late to pull out of firefighting. I'd given leadership my word and was determined to back it up, but by the end of the month, my left knee was twice its normal size and throbbed day and night. Three days before heading north, I opted to get an MRI to understand exactly what I was dealing with.

The tech who conducted my scan had recognized me, and on my way out the door, I asked her if she could tell me anything. Techs aren't supposed to discuss what they see with patients or attempt to analyze images, but she shook her head, and her expression suggested I was in for a rough road ahead.

"Look," she said, "you got a lot going on in that knee."

"What do you mean by that?"

"I mean you won't be doing any running or those triathlons of yours anytime soon."

I'd wanted to tell her that I'd run ten miles before coming to the radiology office but held my tongue because I suspected she was right. I downloaded the results in an Idaho motel room where we stopped to break up the long drive. The official report confirmed multiple tears in the medial and lateral meniscus, a sprained posterior cruciate ligament, general cartilage break-down and arthritis, defects in the lower tip of my femur, a massive Baker's cyst behind the knee, and, to top it all off, a partially torn ACL. In layman's terms, my knee was eight-ways jacked.

2020-05-01 23:16:40 (GMT -00:00)   Page 2/2

1. There is a complex tear in the posterior horn of the medial meniscus. Intrasubstance degeneration in the anterior horn of the medial meniscus
2. There is a tear of the inferior articular surface of the anterior horn of the lateral meniscus. There is also intrasubstance degeneration in the anterior and the posterior horns of the lateral meniscus.
3. There is an osteochondral defect in the medial femoral condyle. There is no free floating fragment
4. Partial tear of the anterior cruciate ligament
5. Sprain of the posterior cruciate ligament
6. Partial tearing of the medial and lateral retinaculum
7. Patella alta
8. Sprain of the quadriceps tendon. Tendinopathy of the patellar tendon
9. Tenosynovitis of the popliteus tendon
10. Suprapatellar joint effusion
11. Popliteal cyst
12. Lobulated cyst surrounding the posterior cruciate ligament
13. Soft tissue edema in the medial aspect of the knee
14. Moderate arthropathy of the knee

MRI report on my left knee, May 2020

The news was deflating. The feeling of an honest day's work is the best feeling I will ever have in my life, and for nearly a year, I'd been looking forward to getting back into the mountains to grind with a backcountry fire crew. We'd blocked off five months and declined all speaking engagements for that period of time, and now, my season looked doomed. As I lay awake that night, Kish reminded me that we still had two weeks before day one of training and that we knew an innovative, thirty-five-year-old sports physio based in Missoula, where we'd rented a studio apartment for the summer.

Casey specialized in working with world-class athletes and was often on the road with a well-known professional tennis player—in fact, we'd met him at a tournament in Rome in 2019—but because the coronavirus pandemic had suspended the tour, he was back home seeing patients and able to work me into his daily schedule. Two weeks obviously wasn't enough time to fix my knee, but I didn't need to be 100 percent. If he could help me get even 10 percent healthier, it might be enough.

Two days later, I limped into Casey's office where 120 milliliters of bloody synovial fluid was pulled out of the knee. Enough to fill multiple vials. It was like watching a blow-up toy get reduced to a wrinkled shell after all the air leaked out, and it was obvious that the joint had very little structural integrity left. My range of motion was freakish. My lower left leg moved like a pendulum, nearly forty-five degrees to either side, while the patella floated like an air-hockey puck.

For the next two weeks, I spent four to five hours a day with Casey for a regimen of massage therapy, range of motion work, and a treatment called "dry needling," which is similar to acupuncture. He stuck me with over two hundred of those things. I was a man-sized pin cushion. We had the knee drained twice more for good measure, and while I submitted to whatever crazy interventions he devised, all I could do was hope.

I hoped something might work. I hoped Casey might crack the skeletomuscular code to heal my wobbly knee. That his needles held the power to not just reduce inflammation but reconnect frayed and torn ligaments and regrow cartilage. More than anything, I hoped that we wouldn't be asked to dig sidehill on a steep slope. I could deal with pain and had enough stability to move straight ahead on flat ground, but lateral movement of any kind, especially on uneven terrain, would be impossible. Unfortunately, Montana is not known for an abundance of flat ground, and as we know, hope is not an anchor point. In other words, I hope you know that I knew I was screwed. But I showed up early the first morning of training, regardless.

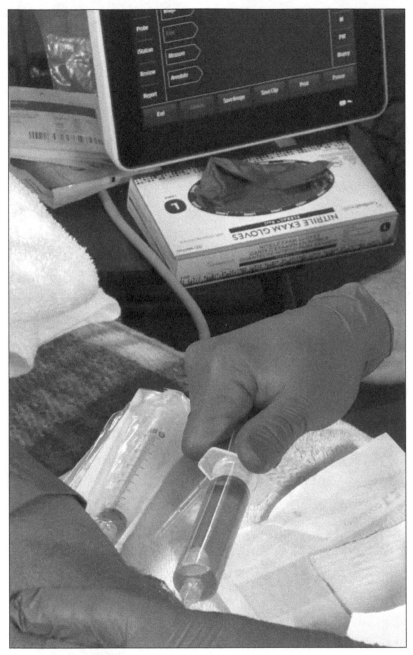

First of many drainings in May 2020

My 2020 fire season ended on an all-night dig. We rucked into the wooded mountains north of Missoula, where I withstood the pain for five hours while I scrambled to find stable footing. I used boulders and logs to support my buckling left leg as I swung at the hard ground with my Pulaski. In the evening, as we approached the top of a slope, I stepped on a slick log cloaked by leaf litter. My left leg went two directions at once, my knee popped, and like one of those Imperial Walkers in the *Star Wars* movies, I collapsed in a contorted heap. In one agonizing misstep, my fate was sealed.

My eyes watered from the pain when the emergency room doc reset my dislocated patella later that night. The orthopedist who conducted MRIs on both my knees the next day said that in his professional opinion, I had the knees of a ninety-year-old man, which only confirmed exactly how I felt. He hinted that knee-replacement surgery was in my near future and instructed me to take several months off. I was in a bad way, and I had to accept that, but just like the night before, I didn't let the news or the pain get in my head for long. Unfortunate situations never last, but I knew that a bad attitude always lingers and can turn any setback into a tailspin.

The only thing more infectious than a good attitude is a bad one. The more you dwell on the negative, the weaker you feel, and that weakness infects those around you. However, the reverse is also true. I knew that if I could control my attitude and redirect my attention, I'd gain control of the entire situation. I was disappointed, but I wasn't surprised that my knee gave out. Now, it was on me to learn what I could from the setback, adapt, and move forward.

It's an unwritten natural law of the universe that you will be tested. You will get smacked in the face. A hurricane will land on your head. It's inevitable for all of us. Yet, we are not formally taught how to handle unexpected adversity. We have sex education, fire drills, active-shooter drills, and curriculum on the dangers of alcohol and drugs, but there is no rug-just-got-pulled-out-from-under-you class. Nobody teaches how to think, act, and move when disappointment, bad news, malfunction, and disaster inevitably strike. All the advice floods in only after we are already lying dazed on the canvas. Which means it's up to you to cultivate your own strategy and have the discipline to practice it.

Mine is simple. No matter what life serves me, I say, "Roger that." Most people think "Roger that," simply means, "Order received." However, in the military, some people infuse ROGER with a bit more intention and define it as, "Received, order given, expect results." When used that way, it is so much more than an acknowledgment. It's an accelerant. It bypasses the over-analytical brain and stimulates action because, in some situations, thinking is the enemy.

I'm not suggesting that you should follow every order like a robot. After you've been knocked down, it's important to take some time to understand what happened and strategize your way forward, but you also must act. If you stay stalled out, sifting through the wreckage, you may find that you've been swallowed by it. We all love comeback stories because they teach us that setbacks have the power to propel us forward to our greatest successes, but your fate depends on your approach. After an injury or failure, your mind wants to either spin out into overthinking or fall back into numbness and complacency, and it takes practice to short circuit that process.

"Roger that" is a ticket back to your life, no matter what happens. You may be laid off, run down, flunked out, cut, or dumped. You could be a stressed-out, bullied young kid, an over-weight veteran with no prospects, or simply handed a pair of crutches and told to sit tight on the sidelines for as long as it takes to heal. The answer is always "Roger that." Scream it out loud. Tell them all that you heard what they had to say and that they can expect your very best in return. And don't forget to smile. A smile that reminds them that you are most dangerous when you're cornered. That is how you respond to a setback. It's the most efficient way to deal with adversity and come out clean.

Casey had heard what happened, and he assumed I'd be demoralized, but when he stepped into his office after lunch, I was already there, doing pull-ups, my knee immobilized in an air cast, my crutches leaning against his back wall. I'd had enough time to digest my situation and had only one question for him.

"Do you think I'll be healthy by the second week of October?" I asked.

"Healthy enough for what, exactly?"

"Moab 240." He looked baffled, so I explained a bit about the race. He thought it was all a joke and turned to Kish to confirm his suspicions.

"He's not even remotely kidding," Kish said.

Casey could see in my eyes how serious I was, so he grabbed my file and read the summary of both MRIs aloud. It was all there. But just as it was with any diagnosis I had ever received, there was a challenge buried in the bad news. Casey missed that, but I didn't.

"Let's not have any expectations," he said. I smiled and nodded.

"Roger that."

Having a target allowed me to strategize and prioritize. It

wasn't just about healing. Whenever something sets me back, I always set a goal, something tangible to shoot for, that keeps me task-oriented and prevents me from being consumed by the sorrow of whatever is going on.

But it's important that your goal isn't too readily attainable. I like to set audacious goals during dark times. Too often, people are convinced that they are challenging themselves by aiming to accomplish something they've done countless times before. I hear it whenever someone comes to me for training advice, which is a lot. Spoiler alert: it rarely goes the way they'd hoped. Recently, someone asked how to best prepare for a half-marathon.

"Why are you running a half-marathon?" I asked. "You're already training, so why not a full marathon?" He tripped over his tongue trying to come up with a satisfying answer, but I already knew why. He was training for something he knew he could do. I'm not picking on him. That's how most of the world operates. Very few individuals step outside the box and attempt to stretch their limits. They rule out the spectacular by default. They put a hard cap on their own performance way before game day. The fact that I'd put Moab out there would keep me dreaming big through the drudgery of rehab, and it also set me up for the possibility of doing something special.

It didn't guarantee it. Not by a long shot. My body would have to respond to all my effort and commitment. I'd have to prove that I could run long distances again in order to make it to that starting line, but if all of that lined up, I would be rewarded with a unique and rare opportunity. That is, to come back from injury and earn redemption in Moab. The fact that I believed that I was capable of that, despite my condition, gave me confidence and strength. Strength that was mine to keep. Strength I could rely on even if it turned out that my rehab went nowhere and it became clear that I couldn't run like I used to. That was my worst-case scenario, and if it happened, I already knew what I would do. I'd set another unreasonable goal and get back to work.

During my long days of rehabilitation, I envisioned what the immediate future might bring, starting with the worst-case scenario and working forward from there. Locking eyes with the worst-case is always my starting point in any endeavor because it removes the fear of failure, prepares me for any and all outcomes, and keeps me leaning net positive from jump.

Whatever happens to us in life, we must aim to keep things net positive. When you have a bad day, it's tempting to call it an early night and try to forget about it, but if you go to bed in the red, chances are you'll wake up that way, and all too often, that type of negativity snowballs. When your entire day is messed up, make sure that you achieve something positive before lights out. You'll probably have to stay up a bit later to read, study, get a workout in, or clean the house. Whatever it takes to go to bed in the black, get it done. That's how you stay net positive on the day to day, and when that becomes automatic, it will be so much easier to see any emotional tripwires coming, which will help you strategize around them.

In Montana, that meant I had to keep an open mind and stay grounded in reality. I knew my goal was far-fetched, and I didn't necessarily expect to be able to finish Moab 240. Maybe I could run fifty miles? Maybe I could knock out one hundred? In this situation, the worst thing that could possibly happen was I don't even start the thing. There was an even better chance that it would be canceled like everything else because of the coronavirus. I could live with all of that because there are always other races, and I knew I would emerge from this experience with five months of intense training and rehabilitation, which could only help me going forward. Two weeks in, I still had no idea when I would be able to run again, yet I remained focused on and worked toward my unreasonable goal, which allowed me to turn all the discomfort and frustration I was feeling into nutrients that primed me for growth.

Meanwhile, the news was impossible to ignore. The first viral wave had swept across the nation, leading to lockdowns, overflowing hospitals, mask mandates, and a general population used to living very comfortable, predictable lives losing their collective grip in the face of tragedy and adversity. Many things in life are masked by circumstance. My weak, degrading knees had been disguised by strong quad muscles that could compensate for the joint's lack of stability, and now, my whole life had been upended.

The coronavirus exposed society's lack of stability. It showed us that national unity is fragile and that the social structures and habits we've relied on can be vaporized at any moment. In the spring of 2020, life had become real, and suddenly, everybody was home and a lot of us were feeling exposed. The unemployment rolls swelled, people were sick and dying, rent went past due, schools were shuttered, and supply chains ground to a halt. That's exposure on a global level. Everything was upside down, and it was scary, frustrating, and unpredictable, and a lot of people did not pass the test. They were caught unprepared. I wasn't.

We all have one thing in common. We are here, stuck in the game of life, often subject to the whims of forces beyond our control, but we never train for it. We dedicate ourselves to external goals, whether they are rooted in fitness or school or work, as if they are isolated events, somehow disconnected from the totality of our lives. When everything we do is an opportunity to get better at the game of life itself. My life and my commitment to do what needs to be done even when I don't want to prepared me for the pandemic, but only because I've come to see everything I've done and been through as training.

I am a student of life. I carry around a notebook. I keep logs. I study all the upswings and down currents of my days as if the final exam is tomorrow. Because we all have an exam tomorrow. Whether we realize it or not, every interaction, each task is a reflection of your mindset, values, and future prospects. It's an opportunity to be the person you've always wanted to be.

You don't have to have survived trauma or become a physical beast to train for life. We've all been challenged physically, emotionally, and intellectually, and we've all failed. Don't be shy about digging through your lost archives. No matter how irrelevant those experiences seem now, they count because they were all dry runs for whatever comes next.

This awareness that everything we do is merely training for the next episode is like a filter that expands your perception. When you get assigned something at work or school that you don't want to do, step into a conflict you didn't see coming, someone close to you gets sick or dies, or a relationship falters, you will see these challenges as new chapters in life's textbook, which you can study to make sure that the next season of loss won't be such a kick in the knees. Not just for you, but more so for the people around you. We all know that training is required to make the cut in competitive sports, get into the best schools, and compete for the most coveted jobs because that's what it takes to be prepared. If the pandemic proved one thing, it's that everyone can be better prepared to handle life's sudden dark twists.

After a month of intense rehab, I went for a three-mile run to evaluate how far I'd come. While my pace was pedestrian, I was shocked at how different my stride felt. I had always had more of a scooting running style, unable to stride it out. But on this first run, my whole body absorbed the impact when my foot hit the ground, not just my knees. That was a major improvement I could build upon, which is exactly what I did.

As always, my ace in the hole throughout this process had been Kish, but her time in Montana had come to an end, so I shifted gears into straight-up monk mode. My whole existence revolved around training, visualization, and recovery. Some of that time I spent with Casey. And while it's a fact that he came up with PT I'd never heard of before—like hitting the VersaClimber with pressure cuffs looped around my legs and utilizing a high-speed muscle-stimulation machine during abdominal and leg workouts—for every hour I spent with him, I put in another five-plus hours on my own.

Most people who attempt to recover from an acute injury see their physical therapist a few times a week for an hour at most, yet they make that therapist their leader and convince themselves that it is the therapist's job to fix them. We can't rely on others to get us to where we need to be. We need more personal ownership and self-leadership. When I was struggling in school, my mom brought in tutors a couple of times. The first time around, it didn't help much because I only cracked my schoolbooks when that tutor showed up once a week. Instead of using her as a guide to help me figure out how to learn better on my own, my tutor became a glorified homework coach. That situation didn't last long, and I fell further and further behind. The second time we hired a tutor, I had my mind set on graduating and passing the ASVAB, and it worked. Not because the second tutor was better, but because I was committed to my own success and put in work on my own.

Casey helped me a lot, but he wasn't my leader. He was a consultant. I was in charge of my own rehabilitation, and I worked at it up to ten hours a day, seven days a week, because I was on the clock. I needed to build strength and rehabilitate in a timely fashion, or Moab would never happen. I tightened up my diet to lose any excess weight and ease the load on my knees. I incorporated heart-rate training for the first time in years. I dipped back into cross-training. I swam, rowed, and spent hours on the Jacob's Ladder and the AssaultBike. I was open to any exercise with a high suck factor that I could maintain for long periods of time while sparing my knees. My sleep was the best it had ever been. And with every workout and each passing day, the dog got hungrier and hungrier. Operation Moab Redemption was on track.

Of course, whenever David Goggins feels like he's got it all figured out, instant karma bites back. I endured bouts of intermittent swelling and continued to have my knee drained. In fact, five days before the race, we drained a baseball-sized Baker's cyst behind my knee because it was inhibiting my newfound range of motion. Yeah, I still had issues, but I certified my knee as "good enough," and on October 7, I toed the line. That was a major accomplishment. As far as I was concerned, I was already in the black, and whatever happened from here would be gravy. Which freed me up to run my tail off.

I was shocked at how good I felt and kept waiting for the wheels to fall off. Around mile seventy, I started to feel a tendon above my left ankle, and while it hurt like hell, I tried not to focus on it. My attention was dedicated to following my blueprint to a T. Around mile 130, I ran out of water during the hottest time of day. It was ninety degrees, I went through one hundred ounces quicker than ever and became dehydrated several miles short of the next aid station. My pace went from brisk to sluggish, and licking my lips wasn't helping a whole lot. While dehydration was a concern, I also had much bigger issues. My new stride put a lot more pressure on my left ankle. It held up well for the first part of the race but had hit its limit, and the pain was no longer something I could ignore or move to the back of my mind. It was loud.

We called ahead, and Kish was able to have water, pickle juice, and electrolytes ready when we arrived at the aid station at around two in the afternoon. I was comfortably in second place, about an hour behind the leader. The only shelter was our support vehicle, and I sat shotgun while I hydrated. Kish placed ice packs under my arms and on the back of my neck, and I placed one in my groin area, all the trigger points that bring the core temperature down quickly. The rest of the crew left us alone. I got so cold so fast that pretty soon, I was jackhammering, and this time I surrendered to it. Kish sensed my concern.

"Something is bothering you," she said, "but I can't help you if you don't tell me what it is." I nodded and took off my left shoe. My anterior tibial tendon, which sits above the ankle joint, was swollen as thick as a rope, and any movement at all felt as if I were piercing my foot with a red-hot blade. The pain was so palpable that even Kish was clenching her teeth when she picked up the phone to call Casey.

I had asked Casey to join the crew because it was obvious that the old blood-and-guts routine I'd relied on for so long wouldn't be enough this time. My forty-five-year-old body was breaking down, and I had a feeling I'd need his expertise somewhere along the way. Trouble was, he was resting back at the crew cabin in Moab and couldn't get to us for an hour and a half. That was on me. I should have made sure he was at every aid station, especially this deep into the race, but it wasn't in the blueprint.

I'd been awake for about thirty-six hours straight by then, and all I could do was close my eyes and try to get some sleep while awaiting his arrival, but between the heat, my ankle pain, my racing heartbeat, and stress from the running clock, I couldn't relax. I kept picturing the race leader scampering ahead like a jack rabbit while I was stuck.

"Thanks for all the rehab, bro. I now have a new stride, and my ankle is jacked," I said with a wry smile. Casey had arrived and was inspecting my foot and ankle from every angle. The joint was partially dislocated, and my tendon was extremely puffy, as if it were getting ready to pop through my taut skin. "Tell me you can fix it."

He set my foot down gently and nodded, his hands on his hips. He had this look in his eye that reminded me of the medics that hang around Hell Week. Those guys are a special breed. They witness a lot of suffering but are programmed never to show sympathy or tell you to quit. Your bone could be coming out of your skin, and they will blow on it, tape it up, and say, "You're good to go." Casey's demeanor was just like theirs, which convinced me that he'd figured something out to keep me moving, but it would be evil, and I would have to suck it up!

"This tendon wants to rupture," he said. That startled me. Kish too. "It's okay. I can prevent the rupture and stabilize it enough that you can continue to run, but it's going to hurt like hell."

For the next hour, he scraped my puffy tendon with a blunt,

metal instrument while I lay back on his portable treatment table wearing blinders. The only way I can describe the pain is that it was so bad, I could only laugh or cry. And I chose laughter.

"Used to be that the only people stupid enough to think that running 240 miles was a good time were White people," I said while Casey dug into my tendon, trying to move the fluid enough to slide my joint back into place. "Then I showed up!

"You all realize I'm choosing to do this, right? That this is my choice! Not only that, I'm paying for it. I paid for this guy right here to fly to Utah to torture me with a blunt instrument in the middle of nowhere!"

The harder Casey scraped my tendon, the louder my howls of laughter became. We are talking out-of-control, breathless belly laughs. Pretty soon, the whole crew was dying.

When I first limped to Casey's table, I'd been pissed off, and the crew looked somber. They had all been excited when I was running with the leader for the majority of the first ninety miles. They'd watched me perform and helped me strategize to maintain my iron grip on second place while I waited for the back half to make my move, only to witness yet another setback. Something almost always breaks down for me. That's no secret, but it's frustrating to find yourself in the same position over and over.

The crew felt bad, but I didn't need or want their sympathy. I couldn't use it. Sympathy has no power. Humor, on the other hand, picks everyone up. It is a huge morale booster. Laughing at yourself and the absurdity of life and your own goofy choices gets the endorphins flowing and the adrenaline pumping. It helped me take the pain and distracted my crew from the fact that the rest of the race would almost certainly devolve into a walk fest. They all thought so because it was obvious that my ankle was seriously injured, and they knew from the tone of my voice and my laughter that I wasn't about to quit.

A person who refuses to quit has a lot of tools at their disposal, and I didn't use humor merely as a numbing agent or a tool of strategic distraction. I used it to lock in even deeper. The more Casey worked on me and the louder my team laughed, the clearer I could see that my race wasn't close to being over.

Keep laughing, I thought to myself. *Wait until you see me on the back half of this course.* Turned out that all that laughter had reawakened the sleeping savage within.

More than three hours after I'd arrived at the aid station, my ankle was back in joint and wrapped in six types of athletic tape to prevent me from flexing it. It was almost like a cast, but Casey assured me that, despite how it felt, it could take some pounding.

"This joint needs to move," he said. "It's gonna hurt, but moving on it is the best thing for it." In other words, Merry Christmas.

After being down for three and a half hours, and now four full hours behind the leader, it was time to see what I could do. As luck would have it, Ms. Kish was next up as pacer. As we left the aid station, Jason, another member of my crew, approached Casey.

"Think it will hold up?" he asked.

"We'll know at the next aid station," Casey said. A few seconds later, I reappeared on the trail below, and Kish could barely keep up. "Or you can turn around and see for yourself."

Prior to the race, Kish selected the very same section she'd enjoyed so much in 2019 for her shift as pacer, and I'd been looking forward to this moment for a year. Of the entire 240-mile course, I'd visualized this section right here far more than any other, and as soon as we were on the trail, I pushed the pace. Four miles in, Kish grimaced, glanced at her smartwatch, and looked puzzled.

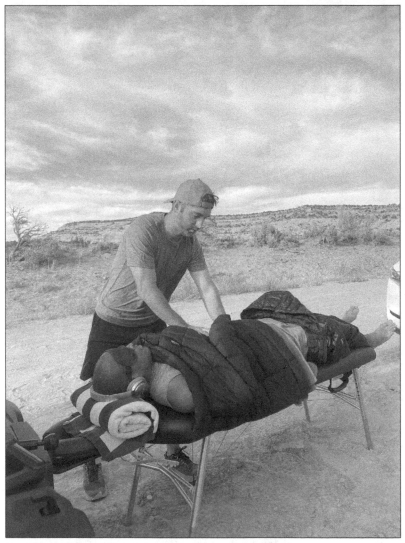

Getting dialed in at mile 140

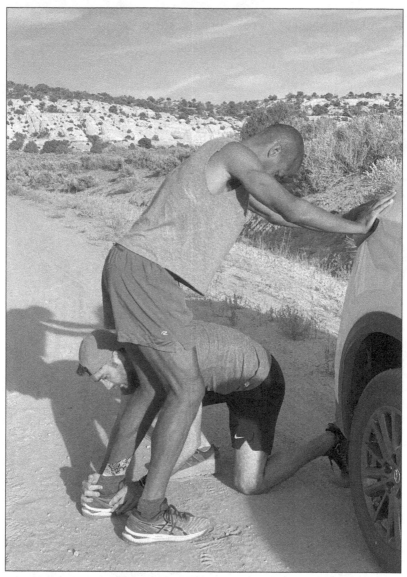

Final ankle adjustments at mile 140

"I don't think we went this fast last year," she said.

"Oh, you noticed?" I asked, smiling to myself. "Call Casey and tell him it's on!"

I accelerated uphill, which took Kish by surprise. As pacer, it was her job to stay with me, and she sprinted to catch up. In fact, to her great displeasure and for the first time in the race, I was running every hill. Finally, when we arrived at the bottom of another incline, she grabbed my arm to stop me.

"Don't you want to walk this?" she asked, breathless.

"Okay," I said, laughing to myself, but before we reached the top, I took off again. Kish is a very good runner, but she wasn't expecting to be in a workout this deep into my race. Especially after all the talk about ruptured tendons. I could see it. I could hear her breath. She started calling out hills well ahead of time. Unless I called for intervals first. Several times, I told her we would run for five minutes and walk for three, only to stretch those five-minute intervals to twenty and then twenty-five minutes. I enjoyed watching her stew in the unknown.

Was I torturing sweet Kish? Yes. Yes, I was. But don't feel too bad for her. I had my reasons, and I know what makes her tick. Kish is extremely warm, refined, and polite, but don't let the smooth taste fool you. Look who she fell in love with. That lady is a thug, just like me. There's some serious dog in that woman, and she does not tolerate any weak sauce.

When we first got together, she kept mentioning how there had always been something missing in her past relationships. No one ever pushed her enough. She was never challenged, and she loves to be challenged. In fact, she'd dogged her exes so hard so many times that during Moab 2019, when she saw me suffering on terrain she handled so easily, I couldn't help but imagine what she might be thinking. And it was mandatory that I earn back any respect that I'd lost in these here hills.

I knew I'd done my job when she finally said, "I don't remember this section being so hard." Once again, I laughed, and laughed out loud.

We finished Kish's section ninety minutes faster than in 2019, and I was only getting stronger, but now, it was time to venture into the high country and tackle the terrain that threatened my life the year before. As the trail pitched up in altitude toward a ridge that loomed like a coiled dragon, I couldn't shake the fear. I was afraid of how my body would react after being awake and running for forty hours. I was terrified that my longtime lung issues would return with a vengeance. I was scared I wouldn't make it.

I'm afraid a lot, but I've learned to flip fear by facing whatever it is I'm scared of head-on. When I first started to face my fears, I was tentative. That's normal, and the emotions and discomfort I felt were proof of how potent this process can be. My anxiety stirred and my adrenaline pumped as my mind edged closer to what I was so desperate to avoid. But within all that energy is a mental and emotional growth factor that can lead to self-empowerment.

Just as stem cells produce a growth factor that stimulates cellular communication, muscle growth, and wound healing in the body, fear is a seedpod packed with growth factor for the mind. When you deliberately and consistently confront your fear of heights or particular people, places, and situations that unsettle you, those seeds germinate, and your confidence grows exponentially. You might still hate jumping off high things or swimming beyond the waves, but your willingness to keep doing it will help you make peace with it. You may even be inspired to try to master it. That's how a kid who was afraid of the water his whole life became a Navy SEAL.

Some people take the opposite path and hide from their fears. They are like villagers terrorized by rumors of a dragon to the point that they cannot leave their own property. They cower, and that dragon, who they have never seen themselves, only gains strength and stature in their minds because when you hide from whatever it is that freaks you out, that growth factor works against you. It will be your fear that grows exponentially while your possibilities become ever more limited.

I had forty miles of steady altitude gain in front of me. That is a lot of time to contemplate last year's breakdown, and quick cuts of me doubled over, begging for breath did flash in my head, but each step up onto another hump of the dragon's spine confirmed my commitment to the task at hand. Until I became the knight who turned up in that village one quiet evening, sharpened my sword, and slayed the dragon.

In 2020, the thin air did not trouble me. My lungs were clear, and I ran so well that my pacers had trouble checking me, but it all came at a cost. A vicious rash had erupted on my butt, my entire left foot was one giant blister, and after lasting for nearly sixty miles, the careful tape job that supported my ankle was unraveling, along with my focus. I was in so much pain, it was difficult to walk, much less run, and impossible to think. Goggins the savage had fled the scene, and it was David who topped out at mile 201 and hobbled into the aid station.

That rash stung so bad I crab-walked to the porta potty without a word. Kish tailed me with a clean set of clothes and an industrial-sized tub of Desitin diaper cream. When she yanked my drawers down, she gasped at the ugly scope of work. My butt cheeks had turned to hamburger meat. They were seeping, but Kish got right up in there and smeared that zinc-based cream wherever it had to go until her hands were covered in my blood. That's true love. Each time she touched the rash, an electric shock of agony zipped up my spine and snapped my jaw shut. For an encore, Casey lanced and taped my blisters and rewrapped my ankle. That didn't feel too good either, but

I was too tired for another comedy show. The entire process took an hour, which was too long, but I didn't mind at the time because I was too deep in the hurt locker to consider anything but survival.

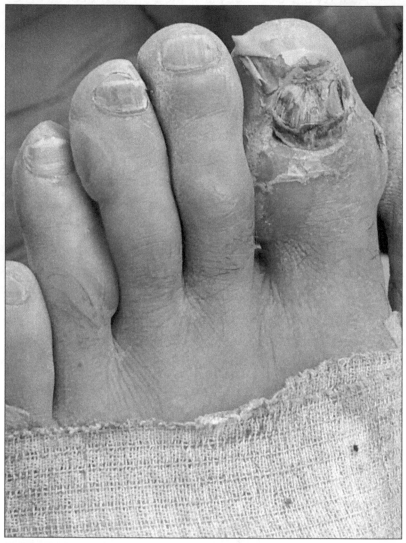

The dogs hurting at mile 201

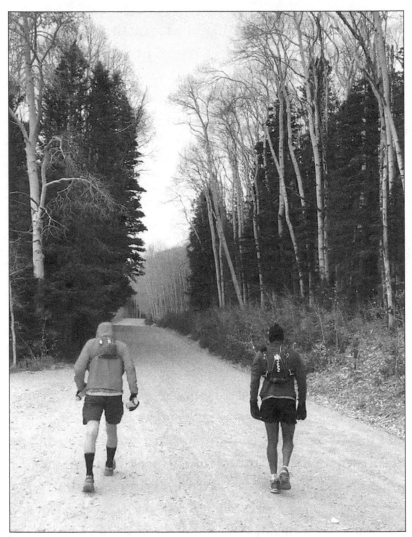
Mike and me heading out at mile 201

The pain was bordering on biblical as my pacer, Mike, and I started out again and scraped along at a zombie's pace. My butt felt like it was being sliced and fileted with rusty razor blades with each step. My blisters burned, and it seemed like it was a matter of time before that tendon in my ankle snapped like a rubber band. Six miles in, we came across a campsite toilet set up by a lake. I lied and told Mike I had to hit the head. In reality, I was desperate to get off my feet. With thirty-three miles left, I'd hit my breaking point, and all I wanted was for this race to be over.

Pain had never stopped me in an ultra race before. Yet, there I was, in a fugue state, ducking and hiding in the outhouse, quaking in my running shoes. That's when Goggins reappeared and found me there. Goggins knew that the only way to deal with pain is to run straight through it, so he knifed David, stuffed him down the toilet, and took over.

From that point on, I performed at a level I didn't think was still possible for me. I used Mike as fuel and raced against him like he was my competitor. I dropped him on a descent. Long, boring, downhill terrain is his only weakness as a runner, and it's my strength. Anything long and boring is my strength, and I put several minutes on him. Mike is a very successful guy. He works in finance in New York City, and he's an accomplished ultra runner. He is not used to being dropped, let alone by someone two hundred miles into a race, and it made him angry.

I slowed down and let him catch up, and when he did, he called Kish to tell her we were running well ahead of schedule, which shocked her because she was at the crew cabin doing laundry and didn't expect to have to be back on course for several hours. Then, he called his wife, who is also an elite runner, and fumed about how I'd dropped him. He wanted me to hear how he felt, and when he hung up, he started barking at me too.

He took my behavior as a "screw you," but it was my respect for Mike that encouraged me to try and drop him. I knew how great a runner and competitor he is, and I wanted to strike a nerve. I was picking a fight with a guy who loves a good fight because I knew it would bring more out of both of us, which is what I needed.

Just as I'd hoped, he took it as a personal challenge. I'd inflicted pain and humiliation on him, and it made him surly enough to serve some right back to me. At that point, Moab 240 disappeared, and it became a seventeen-mile race between two alphas who were throwing down. He went from running and walking to hammering, and it hurt both of us. By that point, I'd covered 220 miles, and he'd run eighty, and we still clocked sub-eight- and then sub-seven-minute miles, and attitudes were everywhere. Somewhere in there, we decided to be friends again, and he looked over at me, mystified.

"I've never seen this before," he said. "You're a freak. You can lift heavy and run like this? Your ankle and knee are all messed up, you're two hundred miles into this race, and you drop me?"

I get that kind of thing a lot from friends and strangers. They read about me taking on incredible challenges and frequently performing at a high level or witness it themselves, and they think I was born for it. That I have some innate quality they lack. Even after *Can't Hurt Me*, many people still feel that way, when in fact, the opposite is true. I was born with birth defects, very few prospects and raised in hell, but I found a way. Mike knew my whole story, but he'd experienced something he'd never seen before. He'd watched me defy my broken body and not just refuse to quit but show out in a way that defied logic.

"I'm not a freak," I said. "I'm just a guy who believes in himself more than most. I am aware of what we are all capable of and that to get there, I have to harness every bit of power and energy I can. Power that is within all of us and all around us. I use your weakness as strength. I use your aggravation as strength. I ignite my competitive spirit with yours to get me moving even faster. Because if I can drop a hard man like you this deep into a race, what does that say about me?"

Mike had gone from surly to giddy by the time we hit the next aid station. Our goal was to get there in seven hours. We arrived in five. I was exhausted from racing him, but there was only an hour and a half of daylight left and sixteen miles still to run, which meant I had to keep it moving. During my rehab in Montana, Casey started to run with me, and he'd impressed me enough that I asked him to take me home.

Barring catastrophe, I had second place locked, but before taking on each new section, I set micro-goals on the fly. The terrain ahead was filled with rolling hills and narrow trails littered with cobbles and boulders. My goal was to keep my average pace faster than twelve and a half minutes per mile. If I did that, I'd finish with the fifth-fastest time ever.

We smashed those splits. Even after the sun dropped and our headlamps came out, we were a pair of speed goats. We bounded from one boulder to the next and flew down the narrow singletrack, past sheer drop offs and the shadows cast by the area's abstract red-rock formations. We clocked a few 6:15 miles. The gravel and dust we displaced flew up like puffs of smoke from our heels. Stars glittered above, and the brightest one was my mythical North Star that led me into yet another state of flow and an entirely new dimension.

Until that moment, I'd considered 2007 to be my athletic peak. I was thirty-three years old back then and chewed up 100-mile races like Kit Kats, but I was not yet the mental beast I'd become at forty-five years old. My 2007 self was a hard-core savage in his athletic prime. That guy would run through cinder block walls, but he was less flexible and aware, less strategic. I'm not sure my younger self would have even considered running 240 miles five days after having his knee drained.

The final section of Moab 2020 was the best I'd ever felt

on road or trail, the fastest I'd ever moved so deep in a race, and when the first city lights twinkled below us, I knew that redemption was mine at last. I crossed the line in a state of euphoria. It wasn't the brand of bliss you may be familiar with. It was the Goggins version: nasty and electric. I practically spoke in tongues as I talked to myself, to my demons, to the mountains, to the dark night sky, and to my North Star.

"You don't know me, son!" I howled. "You don't know me, son!"

The sparse crowd cheered, and my team laughed when I hit the dirt and knocked out twenty-five push-ups because I still could. I'd been in second place most of the race. When I left the mile 140 aid station, I was four hours behind the race leader, but I ran one of the fastest back halves of Moab 240 ever and finished in 62:21:29, just ninety minutes behind the winner. The savage was now in full bloom, and he had an unquenchable thirst.

On the drive home, Kish and I discussed our Thanksgiving plans. We were heading to her family's place in Florida for the holiday, and I told her how back in the day, when I traveled as a recruiter, I used to sign up for any ultra races I could find if they were on the way to where I was going. I called them layovers. She tapped the matrix and found a layover in Maryland the week before Thanksgiving. It was called the JFK 50 Mile. I signed up on the spot and finished in 7:08:26, good enough for twenty-fifth place overall.

Casey had been inspired by his own performance in Utah and met us out there to compete in his first ultra. The final twenty miles were a monumental struggle for him, so after my race was over, Kish and I found him on the course, and I paced him all the way home. Which is how my fifty-mile layover became a sixty-two-miler.

I couldn't have been happier with how both races went. While my joints were sore from the pounding and so much time on my feet, my muscles recovered faster than ever before. I felt as if I were hitting an athletic peak I couldn't have seen coming.

The next day, we flew from Maryland to Florida. On Wednesday afternoon, my phone lit up. It was an old friend gushing about a new event he'd recently heard about, the Across Florida 200. It wasn't a race in the true sense. There was no mass start or centralized logistics team, and it was 100 percent self-supported. It started on the Gulf Coast and utilized roughly 180 miles of trails and dirt roads and twenty miles of tarmac as it slithered like a fugitive python northeast across the state to finish where the Atlantic Ocean meets the shore. Runners had seventy-two hours to complete the course, and nobody had managed to do it yet. Some dude hit 120 miles. Another team made it about fifty miles before packing it in.

Kish had worked hard crewing me in back-to-back races and had been looking forward to the weekend and downtime with her family, so I tried to put the AF 200 out of my mind. But the prospect of running the most ridiculous turkey trot of all time spun in my head like an alien moon. Anytime I closed my eyes, it was there, shimmering like a disco ball, daring me to try.

I'm always looking for more fuel because I do not mesh with this modern age, which has a way of sucking the life force out of me. We all must mentally recharge from time to time. Some people like to golf. Others enjoy watching football on Sundays. I go out in the backwoods and crush myself for several days at a time. This was an unexpected opportunity to fill my mental tank to the brim, and after our Thanksgiving feast, the dog was still hungry for scraps, so Kish and I drove north, and on Friday morning, I tapped the Gulf tideline and started running east.

I ran for two and a half days, past hillbilly hunting caravans and drunken drag racers. I jogged on the shoulders of thrumming highways and beneath buzzing powerlines and bloody sunset skies. I cut through private property and navigated swampy, humid forests home to nearly every wild animal Florida had to offer. We're talking vipers, bears, gators, and twenty different varieties of bloodsucking insects. I swear I saw them all. It was a damn Florida Country Safari!

With about thirty miles to go, in the dead of night, I was running on the side of a busy highway when a cop flashed his rollers and cut me off. I hadn't seen a single Black person since the race began, and given what I had seen of North Florida, I braced for the worst, but that White cop greeted me with a handshake and an eager smile. He was a fan, had been following my progress on Instagram, and was hoping to bump into me. After a few friendly words, he sounded his siren, parted the sea of zipping headlights and brake lights, and escorted me across the road, where Kish had parked and was waiting with hot food. Then, he radioed his buddies. Soon, we had three police cars and four cops standing around us, taking pictures and chopping it up. They were all very polite and respectful.

However, the world being what it is, not five miles later, on that same highway, a beat-up truck crept alongside me. I turned and glanced at the kid in the passenger seat just as he hollered the N-word at me.

I shook my head as they drove on, but his ignorance didn't faze me. That was his problem. In fact, the word he'd hoped would wound me bounced right off me. I was on the verge of running five hundred miles of ultra races in less than six weeks.

That is a monumental output, and the reason I pulled it off is because I am focused on being my best at all times. When you live that way, there is no time to donate to small-town racists or anyone else whose perspective is defined by their narrow minds. At this point in my life, the supposedly offensive, unspeakable word with its dark, violent history has been reduced to a chain of harmless symbols: consonants and vowels that don't mean a thing.

With two miles to go, the heavens opened up. Cool, cleansing rain poured in sheets and buckets and washed my sweat, filth, and blood onto the sandy road.

"The rain god's a punk!" I howled. "I wish it were raining harder!"

I followed that road as it unspooled through the trees until it spilled onto a white-sand beach lapped by the Atlantic Ocean. I had officially run across Florida in less than three days and become the first to complete the AF 200.

I was in the best shape of my life at forty-five years old, and I couldn't wait for 2021. With my North Star lighting my way, I envisioned a career year of shattered personal bests.

With that in mind, the following February, I scheduled an appointment with an orthopedist to discuss the nagging pain I felt in both my knees. I'd heard he offered a new stem-cell treatment that might help, but he suggested surgery instead. It would be a simple arthroscopic clean-up job, he said. He would cut away frayed edges, remove floating tissue and promised noticeable improvement after two to three weeks of recovery.

I agreed, but as surgery approached, I became more apprehensive about it. I'd been through hack-job surgeries before, was running well despite the pain, and didn't want to lose what I had. Yet, whenever I considered the entire picture, I came back to what he told Kish and me in his office. The risk was low enough that there was no downside. We'd all agreed on a simple objective: to clear away the source of my residual pain so I could continue to grind.

The morning of my surgery, February 10, I went for a long run. With at least two weeks of downtime ahead, I needed to get one last one in. Then I showered, shaved, and drove to the hospital. My surgeon met me in recovery. The operation took longer than he'd expected, but he didn't mention complications or alter our rehab-and-recovery plan before I was discharged with not so much as a set of crutches.

For the next several nights, the pain was so bad I became nauseous. I had to use the walls as crutches to get to the bathroom from bed. I could barely put any weight on either knee, and I knew I was not supposed to feel this bad after such a simple procedure. Most people can walk immediately and are back to grinding within two weeks. Something twisted and wrong had to have happened in that operating room, but the doctor didn't say anything. And I sensed something else too. I would never run again.

EVOLUTION NO. 7

As far back as I can remember, I craved a seat at the table. Even when I was a teenager, I knew that one day I wanted to sit at that mythical table among the greats in my field. I suppose you can trace it back to a deep desire for respectability. I desperately wanted to be somebody because I felt like a nobody. That's why I was drawn toward Special Ops at such a young age, and when I realized I was flunking out of school, it's why I was so motivated to change. I knew that I would never arrive at that table unless I took myself and my life more seriously. And yet, as much as I wanted to be among the greats, the decision-makers, the anointed ones, I spent years waiting for a formal invitation.

I don't know how many times I visualized receiving that embossed golden ticket to the dinner I dreamed of, where steak and lobster tail would be served by those who admired and wanted to be near us, but I expected to have to prove something first. I figured if I inserted myself into the proper organization or structure and met the standard consistently, someone would notice me—a mentor or guide—and give me directions to where all the power players gathered. I was not looking to be at the head of their table. I wasn't delusional. I just wanted a seat.

In the meantime, I became one of the waiters who served the elite. Before long, some of my peers, who in my mind weren't as qualified as I was, were seated at the table too. I sucked it up and served them, still hoping that one day I'd be tapped on the shoulder and someone would pull out a chair for me. I wanted so badly to be anointed and validated by my superiors. I wanted to be told, "You have finally arrived, David Goggins. You are now recognized to be one of the best."

Trouble is, that formal invitation rarely arrives, and for me, it never did, but while I waited, I observed my so-called superiors at close range. I watched them work, studied how they presented themselves, and realized that most of them were fairly common people. And I wanted to be uncommon. Because it is the uncommon story, the uncommon leader, that inspires others to seek more of themselves, work harder, and rise to the occasion.

It's no secret that the vast majority of people prefer to be led because it's easier to follow someone else than to break your own trail. Yet all too often, we are led by bosses, teachers, coaches, and powerful officials who wear the rank and title and deploy optimistic speeches, management lingo, and strategies they learned in some university or seminar or from their colleagues at that table in the executive suite but do not inspire us. Perhaps it's because they talk way too much and do far too little. Maybe it's because their own lives are out of control. Whatever the case, over time, it becomes obvious that these men and women who we once admired from afar don't have what it takes to lead themselves, let alone anyone else. Yet when they reject or ignore us, we allow that to limit us and our ability to influence the organization we belong to and the people around us.

It doesn't have to be that way.

Too many people mistake leadership for what happens at the top, in the spotlight, around that mythical table, when some of the most powerful leaders are hard at work in the shadows. They know that opportunities to make a difference in the lives of their neighbors, family, coworkers, and friends are ever-present. They wield massive influence without having to say much, if anything at all, and the first step in becoming one of these unsung heroes is learning how to become a self-leader.

Back in 1996, when I was a twenty-one-year-old airman in a Tactical Air Control Party unit (TACP), I subscribed to the basic definition of leadership like almost everyone else. A leader was the person in charge. The one with the highest rank, the fat salary, and the doting support staff. A leader had the power to hire and fire and make or break entry-level peons like me. I never thought a person who had no particular authority over me would end up being such a major influence in my life. I had no clue that I would soon get a crash course in self-leadership and how it can turn anyone into a powerful example that is impossible for others to ignore or ever forget.

Typically, TACP is the liaison between the Air Force and the Army, and I was stationed at an Army base in Fort Campbell, Kentucky, where the renowned Air Assault School is located. Air Assault is known to deliver "the ten hardest days in the U.S. Army." Nearly half of every class flunks out because it combines hard physical training with intellectual rigor as candidates complete an onslaught of physical evolutions and learn how to sling-load choppers with heavy equipment, such as Humvees and fuel blivets. Everything must be rigged in a precise way to ensure the load will break away upon delivery at the right place and time. As an Air Force guy assigned to Fort Campbell for four years, I knew two things. I was guaranteed to be served orders to attend Air Assault School and that if I didn't graduate with that badge on my uniform, it sent a clear message that I lacked motivation and was an underachiever.

Now, did I prepare as if those orders would arrive at any moment? No, I did not. I had everything I needed to become Honor Man at my fingertips, but I didn't tailor my workouts to Air Assault School. I had access to the obstacle course and the two ruck march courses and never got out there for a single training run. I also failed to crack the books or leverage the guys I worked with who had firsthand knowledge of the sling-load test. There were new Air Assault classes running every month. I could have trained and studied hard, then requested Air Assault School when I was ready. Instead, I waited for those orders to land in my lap, and when they did, I showed up unprepared.

The fun started with a physical test on Day Zero, when candidates must run two miles in under eighteen minutes before completing that hellacious obstacle course made up of rib-crushing wall climbs, a rope climb, and a balance test on a network of beams that lead to platforms as high as thirty feet off the ground. There were so many people there that nobody really stood out, and a good chunk of them failed to achieve the basic benchmarks required to be admitted into the school, but I made it.

Before dawn on Day One, I approached the arches that formed the gateway to the Air Assault campus alongside a man I hadn't noticed the day before. Though it was dark, I could tell he was about my height and not much older than me. Now that we officially belonged to the Air Assault class, whenever we crossed under the arches, we were required to perform a set of "five and dimes." That's five pull-ups and ten elevated push-ups. We would cross beneath those arches several times a day, and we always had to pay the same toll.

We grabbed the bar at the same time. I knocked out the standard five pull-ups, but by the time I'd hit the dirt and finished my push-ups, that guy was still on the bar. I stood and watched him perform far more than five pull-ups. Satisfied, he dropped to his feet, fell forward, and hammered a lot more than ten push-ups. Only then did he report to class. We had a hard day of PT ahead. It would include many more push-ups and pull-ups, and the rest of us were content to meet the standard, hoping we would have enough energy to survive the next ten days, yet this man was ready to smoke himself on the dark early morning of Day One. It was the first time I'd ever seen someone do more than what was required. I'd always thought my job was to meet the standard laid out by the brass, but he was clearly not concerned with what was expected of him or what was to come.

"Who is that guy?" I asked nobody in particular.

"That's Captain Connolly," someone said. Okay, so he was an Army captain, but in the Air Assault class, he had no authority at all. He was one of us, just another student trying to earn his badge. At least, that's what I assumed.

A few minutes later, we lined up for a six-mile march loaded down with thirty-five-pound rucksacks. I was only a year and a half out from running six-minute miles and coming in close to the top in almost every run in Pararescue training. In the run-up to Day One, I'd actually had delusions that once again, I'd be at the front of the pack on all the runs and might even win a few, but I had been measuring myself against the general population. My mind was set on that bell curve where 99.999 percent of the population operates, and when it came to getting after it, I figured I plotted out near the top compared to the rest of the class. Didn't matter that I wasn't 175 pounds anymore and that I'd gained thirty-five pounds from lifting heavy and eating garbage. I still looked strong and fit to most people, myself included. Oh, but I was softening up nicely.

When the instructors yelled, "Go," not everybody went out hard. We had ninety minutes to complete the course, and at least half the class intended to walk a good chunk of it. I planned to run/walk the whole thing, knowing that I would bank time running, which would put me out front. For the first two-plus miles, I was in the lead group of five guys, including Captain Connolly. Most of us were smoking and joking. We were running fairly hard, but we were also ripping on each other, and within twenty-five minutes, I was gassed. The Captain, who had been silent the entire time, had barely started to sweat. While we were wasting valuable energy trash-talking, he was self-contained and dialed in, focused on kicking our collective butts.

Around mile three, the road pitched up into the limestone hills, and the whole group seemed to downshift at once and started to walk as if we shared a common mind. We were breathing heavily, and I knew walking the ups and running the flats and downs would be the best way to finish with a decent time and still have something left in the tank for the next several hours of physical training. Captain Connolly did not downshift. He ran on ahead of us, silent as a ghost. Some of the guys squawked about catching him when he inevitably blew up, but I was certain we wouldn't see him again until the finish line. Captain Connolly was an entirely different animal. He was off the bell curve—an outlier. He was not one of us.

It does something to you when you are running close to what you perceive as your limit (back then, I still topped out at 40 percent) and there is someone else out there who makes the difficult look effortless. It was obvious that his preparedness was several levels above our own. Captain Connolly did not show up to simply get through the program and graduate so he could collect some wings for his uniform. He came to explore what he was made of and grow. That required a willingness to set a new standard wherever possible and make a statement, not necessarily to us, but to himself. He was respectful of all the instructors and the school, but he was not there to be led.

The ruck march ended at the arches, and on our approach, we could all see Captain Connolly's silhouette as he completed pull-up after pull-up after pull-up. Once again, he made a mockery of the standard as the rest of us were content to file our five and dimes. Compared to our peers, our performance was well above average, but after watching Captain Connolly flex, it didn't feel like much. Because I knew that while I had been fine with just showing up, he'd prepared for the moment, attacked the opportunity, and showed out.

Most people love standards. It gives the brain something to focus on, which helps us reach a place of achievement. Organizational structure and atta' boys from our instructors or bosses keep us motivated to perform and to move up on that bell curve. Captain Connolly did not require external motivation. He trained to his own standard and used the existing structure for his own purposes. Air Assault School became his own personal octagon, where he could test himself on a level even the instructors hadn't imagined.

For the next nine days, he put his head down and quietly went about the business of smashing every single standard at

Air Assault School. He saw the bar that the instructors pointed to and the rest of us were trying to tap as a hurdle to leap over, and he did it time and again. He understood that his rank only meant something if he sought out a different certification: an invisible badge that says, "I am the example. Follow me, and I will show you that there is more to this life than so-called authority and stripes or candy on a uniform. I'll show you what true ambition looks like beyond all the external structure in a place of limitless mental growth."

He didn't say any of that. He didn't run his mouth at all. I can't recall him uttering word one in ten days, but through his performance and extreme dedication, he dropped breadcrumbs for anybody who was awake and aware enough to follow him. He flashed his tool kit. He showed us what potent, silent, exemplary leadership looked like. He checked into every Gold Group run, which was led by the fastest instructor in that school, and volunteered to be the first to carry the flag.

When the sling-load test came around, I thought that might be his kryptonite. I was hoping that he was just a physical stud, a freak of nature. I wanted to find a flaw in him because it would make me feel better about myself. But when the instructors asked for a volunteer to be the first to take a test that half the class would fail, he didn't raise his hand or say anything out loud. He simply stepped forward to be tested on helicopters, reach pendants, sling sets, proper rigging, and inspection before anyone else. He aced that too.

He won every last physical evolution, was at the top of the class on each of the exams, and raised the level of the entire group. We all wanted to be more like him. We wanted to compete against him. We used him as a measuring stick, as someone we could emulate, because he gave us permission to go beyond the standard. Thanks to him, I volunteered to carry the flag on one of the Gold Runs, and to this day, it is one of the hardest runs I've ever completed. Without the use of your arms, it's impossible to generate the same power and momentum, and that flag feels like a parachute tugging you backward. However, I was nowhere near his physical condition, and when the twelve-mile ruck march came around on Day Ten—our final test in Air Assault School—all I could do was watch him disappear into the distance as he shattered the Air Assault record for the fastest twelve-mile time ever.

I graduated mentally and physically exhausted but felt almost nothing when I was awarded the wings I thought would anoint me as a made man around Fort Campbell. I was still too puzzled and irritated by Captain Connolly's level of effort, which felt almost confrontational. It wasn't a lot of fun to be around him, yet I relished every second. He made me uncomfortable because he exposed my lack of dedication to giving my best effort each and every day. Being around people like that forces you to try harder and be better, and while that is a good thing, when you are inherently lazy, what you really want are some days off. The Captain Connollys of the world don't give you that option. When they are in your foxhole, there are no days off.

His conditioning was clearly off the charts, and I'm not talking about the physical aspect alone. Being a physical specimen is one thing, but it takes so much more energy to stay mentally prepared enough to arrive every day at a place like Air Assault School on a mission to dominate. The fact that he was able to do that told me it couldn't possibly have been a one-time thing. It had to be the result of countless lonely hours in the gym, on the trails, and in the books. Most of his work was hidden, but it is within that unseen work that self-leaders are made. I suspect the reason he was capable of exceeding any and all standards consistently was because he was dedicated at a level most people cannot fathom in order to stay ready for any and all opportunities.

Those who have not learned to self-lead show up to their lives like I did Air Assault School. They don't prepare or have a plan of attack. They wait, get shotgunned into something—a school, a job, a physical test—then wing it. Think about how much information is out there on the internet. Any place you want to build your skills, from boot camp to Harvard Business School, from EMT certification to an engineering degree, is described online in granular detail. You can study the prerequisites and start on the coursework before you are even admitted. You can prepare as if you are already there so when the time comes and you do land that opportunity, you are ready to smash it. That's what a self-leader does, no matter how busy their lives are. Not because they are obsessed with being the best, but because they are striving to become their best.

Self-leaders rarely rest. In the heat of battle, they become dolphins who sleep with one side of their brain on alert and one eye always open so they are ready to outsmart, outswim, or battle their predators and they are awake enough to float back to the surface and take another breath. In order to sustain that amount of energy output, self-leaders return again and again to the organizing ideals of their lives. They live for something bigger than themselves, and because of that, their lives swell and glow with an energy that others can feel. It can also start a chain reaction that challenges and awakens people to the untapped power coiled within themselves. The power that they are wasting with each passing day.

Setting an example through action rather than words will

always be the most potent form of leadership, and it's available to all of us. You don't have to be a great public speaker or have an advanced degree. Those things are fine and have their place, but the best way to lead a group is to simply live the example and show your team or classmates, through dedication, effort, performance, and results, what is truly possible.

That's where I'm at now. Thanks in part to the example Captain Connolly set and because I was aware enough to recognize that he was a rare breed and humble enough to learn from him. However, as you know, the transformation didn't take right away. Sadly, once Air Assault School was over and Captain Connolly was out of my life, the spark faded, and I fell back into my old ways. While I never stopped thinking about that ten-day experience, I didn't have it within me to self-lead just yet. I should have taken the lesson from those ten days and applied it to the next fifty years of my life. I should have imagined Captain Connolly watching me each and every day. Believe me, if you think you're being watched, you live differently. You're more detailed and squared away. That's not how it went for me. It would be another three years of slippage before I exhumed the Connolly files from my personal archives and studied them to become a self-leader.

Two years in the SEAL Teams was all it took to realize that nobody was going to show up to coach or guide me to my seat at the table, but by then, I wanted off the bell curve. I wanted to make my own opportunities and eat alone at my own table. I wanted to become an outlier.

I went on to beat Captain Connolly's twelve-mile ruck-march time, which had been tattooed on my brain for six years, while doing an eighteen-mile ruck march at Delta Selection. I did it on a much harder course with a heavier pack, and for the first twelve miles, I imagined that he was still out there in front of me, dropping breadcrumbs, daring me to exceed the standard he set years ago. He was the first one to show me how to do more with less and that it was not just possible to dig deeper but mandatory if you are striving to be your best self. When I eclipsed his time, I realized I was no longer chasing Captain Connolly. From then on, every school, course, race, or record I took on became an arena for my own self-development.

When you live like that, you are usually far beyond the influence of parents, teachers, coaches, or other traditional mentors and their philosophies. In order to stay humble, you'll need to make sure you are living up to your own code. A lot of great organizations have inspiring mission statements. Elite military units are built around an ethos or creed that defines how their men and women are supposed to conduct themselves. Each time I arrived at a new school or endeavored to join a new Special Operations unit, I studied and memorized the ethos or creed, and those words never failed to move me and most of my peers, but it's human nature to become complacent. No matter how powerful the organizational ideals, even well-meaning people who love what they do—especially those with seniority—will lack the mental endurance to live the creed on the day to day. And if most people within an organization don't truly follow or adhere to the founding principles, then what are they really worth? So, I took my own oath to self:

I live with a Day One, Week One mentality. This mentality is rooted in self-discipline, personal accountability, and humility. While most people stop when they're tired, I stop when I am done. In a world where mediocrity is often the standard, my life's mission is to become uncommon amongst the uncommon.

We all owe it to ourselves to stand for something. Principles give us a foundation—solid ground we can trust and build on as we continue to redefine what's possible in our own lives. Sure, some will be put off by your dedication and level of effort. Others will call you obsessed or think that you've gone crazy. When they do, smile and say, "I'm not crazy. I'm just not you."

Don't rely on some other group's ethos or company's mission statement to be your guide. Don't walk around aimlessly trying to find purpose or fit in. Mine your core principles, and come up with your own oath to self. Make sure it is aspirational and that it challenges you to strive and achieve, and live by it every day.

When everything gets murky and twisted and you feel alone and misunderstood, revisit your oath to self. It will ground you. At times, you will need to revise your oath given the shifting priorities that arise with life changes, but don't water it down. Make sure it is always strong enough to serve as your daily compass as you navigate life and all of its challenges. Living by this oath—your oath—you will never need anyone else to lead you. Because no matter what happens, you will never be lost.

Who will you become and what do you want to stand for? Are you ready to be the standard? If you are willing, share your oath to self. #OathToSelf #SelfLeadership #NeverFinished

CHAPTER EIGHT

PLAY UNTIL THE WHISTLE

Six days after surgery, my knees hadn't improved, and I could barely move at all. I had an appointment on the books to check in with my surgeon, who took one look at my swollen knees and decided to drain them. Instead of synovial fluid, he pulled seventy-five mL of dark-purple deoxygenated blood out of my right knee and thirty mL from my left. Ten days later, the swelling had returned, and he had to drain both knees again. I could tell by the look on the doctor's face that the pain I was in and the persistent swelling were not what he'd expected. Something was truly wrong. While he gave me the third round of platelet-rich plasma (PRP) injections, hoping that might jump-start my healing process, he offered the first clue of what had actually happened in that operating room.

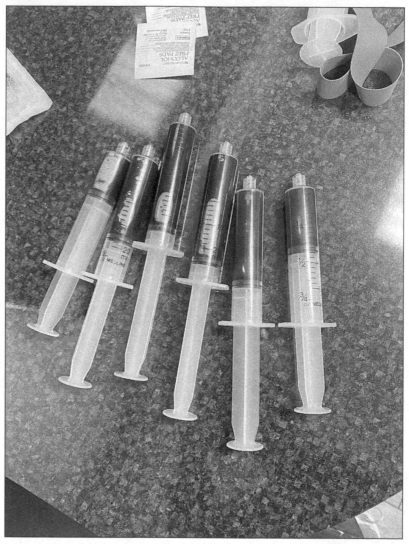

The deoxygenated blood drained from my knees post-surgery was alarming.

I'd gone in for a simple clean-up job on the meniscus, the pad of cartilage that acts as a shock absorber between the tibia and the femur (the shinbone and the thigh bone), but when he attempted to trim the cartilage, his instrument failed. My meniscus and the articular cartilage that clung to the ends of my bones were too thick and tough. He said this was due to

Wolff's Law, a phenomenon discovered by a nineteenth-century German surgeon who found that when an increased load is placed on bones over time, those bones will become denser and much stronger. That sounds like a good thing, but in the knee, it can lead to deterioration or irregularities in the cartilage, which cause arthritis. In my case, the meniscus layer of padding between the bones wasn't thick and smooth like a rubber mat, it was gnarled and twisted like bark and rough like mortar. And the articular cartilage was just as tough. Instead of cutting easily, it was near bulletproof. My torqued connective tissue literally broke the surgeon's high-dollar medical shears.

"Even your cartilage learned to stay hard," he joked.

I didn't laugh much because these were details I should have heard in recovery instead of over two weeks later. That bothered me. However, I couldn't help also feeling a perverse sense of pride. There had been so many times in my life when I felt injured or sick during an intense physical evolution but refused to quit, which forced my body to become the great compensator. I have adapted to deal with several medical conditions over the years—some I'd inherited, others I'd acquired—to complete dozens of strenuous, multi-day feats of endurance. In my doctor's befuddlement, I saw medical proof of that forced compensation. I'd put a heavy load on my bones for so long they had grown dense as stone and transformed my cartilage into cement that was almost impossible to cut through. But, after several failed attempts, the doctor did manage to cut through it.

While recognizing my body's compensation for what it was, a physiological adaptation that enabled me to continue to grind at a high level, he still used a cookie-cutter approach to the surgery. My knees were undeniably damaged prior to the surgery, but I could still function with them. Just a few hours before being wheeled into the operating room, I had run ten miles. Now, two weeks later, I'd limped to a stationary bike at the gym hoping to break a sweat and lasted twenty-two minutes before the pain overwhelmed me. I went from the Moab 240 to running across the state of Florida to twenty-two minutes on an exercise bike.

I returned again to the doctor's office a full month post-surgery, and when I told him how much anguish I was in and how little mobility I had, he downplayed it and in the next breath casually informed me that during the surgery, he'd drilled into one of my bones. At no point during the run-up to surgery had he ever mentioned that as even a remote possibility, and despite seeing me in recovery and twice since then, he had never mentioned that he had drilled two small holes into my left femur. Which was strange because that is not a procedure a doctor is likely to forget.

He said that after removing most of the cartilage in my left knee, he wanted to tap my bone marrow so it would leak out, puddle up, and create a clot that over time is thought to mimic the padding provided by an intact meniscus. He also mentioned that at some point during the surgery, he'd cleared the OR of anyone who was not a vital part of the process. This revelation didn't make me proud. It angered me. I have had several major surgeries in my life, and I'd never received important and unexpected details piecemeal. Surgeons are trained to explain the surgery at the earliest opportunity, but this guy wasn't playing by those rules.

Starting on the day after surgery, there were several times Kish wanted to reach out and ask the surgeon to explain my level of pain and immobility because they were way beyond the expectations he'd laid out. I felt the same way but did my best to control my emotions and avoid hitting the panic button. On the way home from his office after learning about the holes he drilled, however, my anxiety spiked.

That evening, Kish and I did some investigating, and what we read online was unsettling. From what I gathered, it seemed that he'd given me some type of microfracture surgery and never said a word about it. After several sleepless nights, I texted the doctor at around five in the morning and told him I needed some answers, straight up. To my surprise, he replied right away and continued to reiterate that the knees were only going to get better now that they'd been cleaned up. I challenged him on the microfracture procedure. He said a microfracture surgery has a minimum of five holes, he'd "only" drilled two, and that they "should" be filled in by this point. He said pretty soon I'd be back to running like I always had and that nothing would hold me back. I'd had a hunch that this doctor wasn't telling me the full story, but that text exchange confirmed it.

I could no longer trust him. No matter how pure his motives may have been, he'd made questionable, unilateral decisions, performed poorly, left me bone-on-bone, and then fed me unsettling details bit by bit. There was no excuse for any of it.

On March 17, I stepped onto a treadmill for the first time since surgery. I was at physical therapy, and the staff didn't know it yet, but I'd already decided it was my last day. My right knee was feeling a bit better. My left felt much worse than it did before surgery and was collapsing on the medial side. The therapists who had been monitoring my progress were affiliated with my surgeon, and despite my pain, they wanted to see me jog it out for five minutes. I ran for forty-two.

Not because it felt good. Every step hurt, but I kept going because I knew this would be my last run for the foreseeable future, maybe forever, and considering how central running had been in my life for so long, five minutes didn't feel like enough of a farewell. Five grinding miles of agony had more meaning, and when it was over, I powered down the treadmill, stepped gingerly to the floor, and hobbled right out the door.

As I drove home, I felt conflicted between my commitment to remaining patient enough for the great compensating machine to do its work yet again and my fear that it really was all over this time. Despite some of the voices around me that had already accepted my demise as gospel, I didn't want to believe that. I couldn't. Because ever since I decided to not be fat anymore, my whole life has been wrapped around my physical being. While mindset has always been number one for me, I achieved my mindset through physical training and monumental physical challenges that provided an immediate return on investment. That is not the only way to become mentally tough, but it does happen faster when you run thousands of miles, swim long distances in cold water, or do thousands of pull-ups. When you invest that volume of pain and suffering in yourself, it will produce mental toughness.

In other words, my life and my sense of self, from the time I was twenty-four years old until the day of surgery, were built on training and competing hard to become mentally strong. And they were taken from me in ninety minutes. Not by accident or freak injury, but by one doctor who failed to live up to his Hippocratic oath: first, do no harm. I know it was unintentional, but there was major harm done.

I couldn't sweat out the stress, so it was difficult for me to process all the emotion and frustration. There were times that even I wanted to surrender to self-pity. I was tired of Goggins, tired of always fighting the fight, and while I abhor excuses and excuse makers, when I checked myself in that mirror each morning and every night, I told myself the clean truth. *It's over.* *You can't do it anymore.* And I found some comfort there.

I felt like a quarterback at the line of scrimmage reading the defense and clocking nothing but pass rushers with blood in their eyes. The linemen, linebackers, and defensive backs would outnumber and easily overwhelm my blockers, sprint around the edge, bull rush inside, and the pocket would collapse. Unless I averted disaster before it struck. I had to call an audible—yell out a new play at the line of scrimmage loud enough for my whole squad to hear—but as I leafed through the playbook in my mind, I couldn't find any workable solutions.

It's not like this was new territory for me. I'd been facing steep odds and calling audibles all my life, but this was the biggest of them all. When your entire being is rooted in a particular way of life and it gets taken from you, what is the proper play call?

As restless and frustrated as I was, I knew patience was the only play for now. Sometimes, the best thing the quarterback can do is throw an incomplete pass, avoid losing any more ground, stop the clock, and regroup. While I believed my knee was as good as it was going to get, I still wanted to give it time to see if the pain would ease or my stability would improve at all, so it was not the time to tinker. As devastating as it was to go from running over two hundred miles a pop to not being able to walk down a flight of stairs without my left knee collapsing, I had to avoid the temptation to evaluate my situation on the daily and weekly. Instead, I panned back and attempted to see it all with a wide-angle lens.

The summer firefighting season was shot, and I wouldn't be running again anytime soon, which meant I didn't have to scramble for an immediate solution. 2021 was a wash. It was all about next summer and the following season. That reassured me because it meant that there was plenty of time left on the clock. I didn't have to score or even move the ball right away. I just had to watch and wait. I decided to wait a full ninety days (from the day of the surgery) to give my body time and hopefully—there was that word again—compensate for the surgeon's poor judgment and errors. However, when those ninety days were up, nothing had changed. That all-out blitz was still coming for me, and the time for waiting was over. I needed to call a play.

For the next three days, Kish and I parked ourselves at the kitchen table and scoured the internet. We skimmed peer-reviewed studies, medical journals, hospital websites, and physician bios and found that microfracture surgery was usually the last resort for meniscus problems, and when that didn't take, joint replacement was the logical next step. Joint replacement is a type of amputation. The edges of your shin and thigh bones are cut away to accommodate the artificial knee. I was not near ready to go there.

Then, on day four, at exactly the same time, Kish and I happened upon an article featuring the work of a world-class surgeon at the Hospital for Special Surgery in New York City. Dr. Andreas Gomoll was one of the few surgeons in the United States capable of conducting meniscus and cartilage transplants to heal knees so far gone that almost any other orthopedist would consider them candidates for joint replacement. This was the audible I'd been looking for.

According to what we read, a meniscus transplant worked far better than microfracture surgery. It not only reduced pain and restored functionality and quality of life, it might even allow me to get after it to the level I was used to. That mattered to me because I still had unfinished business.

I'd been carrying around the same lofty goal since 2014. It

promised all the physical and psychological demands of Special Operations and was fueled by the same valorous spirit, but whenever I got close to it, the opportunity slipped through my fingers. I wanted to become a smokejumper.

Smokejumpers are airborne wildland firefighters. They parachute into the backwoods to put down fires before they become raging infernos and make world news. My pursuit of smokejumping is the reason I got into wildland firefighting in the first place. After years of frustration, I finally had an opportunity to join a smokejumper crew in Montana back in 2020, but my knees weren't willing to cooperate, and after my failed surgery in 2021, I could only assume that smokejumping would remain out of reach.

On June 7, I met with Dr. Gomoll in New York. He evaluated the MRI scans and took some X-rays of my bowlegged left leg, and my misalignment shocked him. The degeneration in my knee was more severe than he'd anticipated. "I have no idea how you were able to run a mile on those knees," he said. "Let alone fifty, one hundred, two hundred miles."

Dr. Gomoll knew how far I'd traveled to come see him, but as much as he wished he could help, I wasn't a viable candidate for a meniscus transplant because my knee was too far gone. He offered up an unloader brace that might relieve some of my pain but knew it wasn't much of a solution because nobody wears a bulky brace twenty-four hours a day, and a brace alone would not give me my life back.

There wasn't much left to say. He lingered in silence and absorbed my obvious disappointment. It wasn't simply that I was in pain or couldn't work out. I would also have to swallow the fact that the hard-core jobs I'd always admired and strived for were no longer for me. He turned to leave, but when he was halfway out the door, he stopped cold and looked back.

"Hey, try the unloader brace for a couple of months," he said, "and if it helps, there may be one other option we can discuss."

"I would appreciate it if we could discuss it right now," I said. I was desperate for any flicker of possibility at that point. Apprehensive, he nodded, sat down across from me again, and explained an uncommon procedure that isn't taught much anymore known as a high tibial osteotomy, or HTO. It's a surgery that realigns the knee joint to relieve pressure and pain, but to achieve that, he would have to saw into my tibia, open up a five-millimeter wedge to create a gap in the bone, and then screw in a tapered metal plate to cover the gap, which would eventually be filled in with new bone tissue.

"By no means is this a slam-dunk fix," he said, "which is why I hesitate to bring it up." He went on to explain that the outcome had a lot to do with the patient and how determined they are during rehabilitation, but he knew my background and wasn't worried about that. He was reluctant because he knew that both of us could do everything right and my body still might not react well to the procedure. Some knees cannot be helped, and until he was in the operating room, he couldn't say for sure if mine was one of them. "Sometimes, the surgery falls short of solving the problem, and the last thing we want to do is make things worse."

"Definitely not," I said. "But say the surgery is a success, what would that mean for me?"

"Depending on how long it takes for you to recover, eventually, you would have very few, if any, physical restrictions."

"I'm in," I said.

He looked taken aback. Evidently, most people don't leap at the chance to have him saw into their shin bone.

"I still think you should try the brace first."

"You say if this works, I could do anything?" I asked.

"Almost. Everything short of jumping out of planes, I suppose." I paused to digest his statement. At first, it felt like another knife to the gut, but it wasn't definitive. He supposed jumping out of planes would be off-limits, but he did not know me.

"Okay," I said, smiling. "No jumping out of planes. But Dr. Gomoll, you are one of the top guys at the best orthopedic hospital in the United States, and in your professional opinion, you don't see any other options for me?" He blushed slightly at my assessment of his skills. He had a humility about him that I appreciated.

"If you are committed to reclaiming what you've lost," he said, "then I think this is the best choice for you, yes."

Some would look at those odds and consider resorting to an uncommon, painful surgery without a guaranteed outcome a massive risk. I suppose it boils down to what you can and can't live with. A lot of people can live with a lot of mediocrity. Not only can they live with it, they are actually content in it. Well, Merry Christmas to them, but that does not work for me. Oh, I wanted to rest too, but not just yet. If there was even a chance that this was going to get me where I needed to go, then it wasn't even a choice at all.

"Okay then, doctor," I said. "Break the leg."

I had the surgery on June 30 and spent two nights in the hospital and another week in a New York City hotel room. How did I feel? Like someone had just sawed into my leg! When I attempted to stand, the pain level was a ten out of ten. The blood would rush to where that plate was screwed in, leaving me wincing and lightheaded. I scuttled around on crutches and had to shower while sitting in a chair. I iced and relied on electronic muscle and bone stimulation several times a day and did some basic physical therapy exercises while lying in bed.

My flight home was nothing short of excruciating. Agony rolled through me in waves. I broke into a sweat and was borderline delirious as I thought back to my last meeting in Dr. Gomoll's office before we left town.

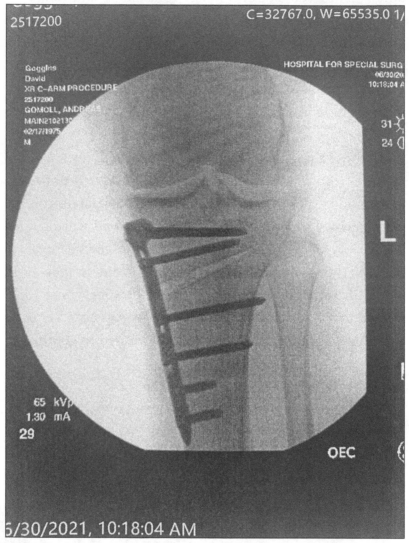

Nothing short of breaking my leg was going to fix my alignment issues.

"The realignment was a success," he said, smiling and pointing at my latest X-ray. I was no longer bone on bone.

Up until that moment, he'd been hesitant to promise too much. I'd managed my expectations too. In the last days before surgery, I'd read countless articles, message boards, and forums on HTO recovery, and, to say the least, they were not encouraging. Most people took three to six months to walk normally. One article sang the praises of a runner who defied the expectations of doctors to complete a marathon eighteen months after his HTO procedure. For me, he became the gold standard. While running a marathon is no easy feat under any circumstances, it was nothing compared to what I would have to do in order to become a smokejumper. If that was even still possible. At my age, every lost fire season is a crucial missed opportunity, and I'd had to sit out the last two. The odds against me were astronomical.

But now that Dr. Gomoll seemed convinced that I was on a different trajectory, I could not help but conjure scenes of smokejumper training. The film was grainy and in black and white, but the soundtrack was familiar. It was the brassy hum of "Going the Distance," and it played on a loop.

"How long before I can start training?" I asked.

"While your knee isn't an issue, the surgery site is. That will take some time to heal. But in a few weeks, you can probably go for a little spin on an exercise bike."

"A little spin," he said. I got through the rest of that flight with visualization. I saw myself wobble to a stationary bike on those damn crutches. I watched the wheels turn and puddles of sweat gather beneath the crank as I spun for hours.

On July 15, just over two weeks after my surgery, that vision became reality. I could barely get my leg over the seat and didn't channel much power into the pedals. Anytime the leg hung loose, it would throb, as if the plate itself came with its own beating heart. Each pedal stroke was another reminder of how bad my knee still was. It was so painful I couldn't help wondering why I was putting myself through it. I lasted thirty minutes. That doesn't sound like much, but it was a monumental first step. The question now became *Can I dial it up?*

Almost nothing in life is constant. Conditions and circumstances are perpetually in flux like the winds and the tide, which is why my mind is never fixed. I tack and adjust, forever searching for my new 100 percent. Age, health, and the responsibilities we carry can be limiting. That doesn't mean we should give in to those limitations or use them as excuses to let ourselves or our dreams go, but we can acknowledge them, as long as we are committed to finding out what we can still do given those limits—whether they be temporary or indefinite—and maximizing that.

When most people undergo major surgery, they relax into the recovery time the doctor lays out. They accept their six- to eight-week vacation from the grind or their six to twelve months of leave. Before I was discharged from HSS in New York, I wanted to know precisely when I could get back into the gym and how hard I could push it. This felt like my last shot, and the stakes were too high to rely on a professional physical therapist. I know my body better than anyone and didn't want any naysayers in the foxhole. The fate of my recovery and my future would be on me, and that kept me thinking proactively.

Every day, thousands of people wake up to a life defined by newfound limitations that are difficult to accept. Maybe they've been diagnosed with a terminal disease or suffered a spinal injury. Could be they lost a limb or are suffering from PTSD. More often, the shifting circumstances are not nearly so dire.

Sometimes, it's good news that changes the equation. Maybe you are a new parent or landed a lucrative gig that demands ten- to twelve-hour workdays. Could be you recently got married, which means you have to consider more than just your own goals. No matter the variables, your new 100 percent is out there waiting for you to find it.

The thing is, most people don't want to. Because whenever you're trying to find your new anything, it means you're not who you used to be, and that can be depressing enough to give up the search. Some people use their new circumstances to dial down their effort level instead of adjusting their approach and still giving it their all to achieve their goals. You've got to work with what you have. I couldn't run or ruck, but that didn't mean I was out of the fight.

No matter what you are dealing with, your goal should be to maximize the resources and capabilities you do have. If you've suffered a freak injury or received a diagnosis that changes everything, what does your new maximum effort level look like? A lot of people bide their time and wait to see what happens next, but a year or two later, they find they are still waiting. With every unfortunate turn in life, no matter how heavy the weight, you have to be committed to pushing back against that pressure with effort. No matter your age, abilities, disabilities, or responsibilities, we must all stay committed to finding our new benchmarks. Because not only does that keep your mind engaged and your demons at bay, you actually might achieve things the old you never could have conceived.

I've never been a faster runner than I was at nineteen years old. Back then, I could blaze a mile and a half in 8:10, but that kid would have laughed if you had asked him to run fifty miles at one time, much less 240. Of course, at forty-six and with a metal plate in my tibia, Moab 2020 felt like a lifetime ago. Prior to the surgery, Dr. Gomoll explained that it was unlikely that I would ever run another 100-mile race again and that medical clearance to run at all was TBD. That did not deter me. I would simply have to find another way to train hard.

Ironically, on June 1, before I even knew who Dr. Gomoll was, I signed up for The Natchez Trace 444, a long-distance bicycle race held in early October. I didn't think I would be healthy enough to compete in it. But I knew running wasn't an option, so it made sense to set imposing cycling goals. When Dr. Gomoll casually suggested the stationary bike, cycling became my anchor point. I latched onto it with a white-knuckle grip and started climbing.

It was not easy. Each morning, as I grabbed my crutches, I felt like I was twenty-four years old and 297 pounds again trying to run just one mile. My leg was badly swollen. Every pedal stroke was torture. The resistance was still very low, but the anguish made me sweat. I wanted to quit a hundred times but refused to give in. Like the fat David from long ago, I was worried if I stopped I might never start again.

For a week, every ride began just like that, but instead of dialing it back, I upped my output. I was still on crutches, mind you. I was non-weight bearing for four weeks and on crutches for six, but I'd ride sixty minutes every morning and another twenty minutes in the afternoon as part of my rehabilitation program. My leg muscles were already getting stronger, and my resting heart rate was starting to drop. All of this represented progress, but those fledgling workouts and my two hours of stretching and range of motion work weren't enough to convince me that I'd be ready to ride four hundred-plus miles by the first week of October. To stop the creep of negative thoughts, I occupied my mind.

Mental and physical fitness have always been intertwined for me, and though I'd missed two consecutive fire seasons, I decided to use my rehab time to gain more knowledge and skills in the event that my body bounced back enough to where even if I couldn't smokejump, I could at least fight fires. One skillset that is attractive to a lot of fire departments is the Advanced EMT certification, but because of my travel schedule, I'd never been able to take the course. This was the perfect time, and I found an accelerated course not far from my place that was about to begin. After I signed up, I dug my old EMT textbook out of my closet, turned to page one, and refreshed my basic knowledge. As far as I was concerned, class was already in session.

As always, my packed calendar worked to my advantage. Each activity fed into the next in a synergy of self-betterment. I had hours to study the human body and learn how to save lives, and I hadn't spent this much time on a bike of any kind since I was training for RAAM in 2009.

During my morning rides, I thought back to those long, peaceful days on the bike. Although running is what I'm known for, I'm actually a better cyclist. Yet, before I could seriously consider racing in October, I needed to get off the stationary bike. In mid-August, four weeks after my first thirty-minute ride, I called Dr. Gomoll and asked if he'd clear me for some road miles.

"How long do you plan to ride?" he asked.

"Four hundred and forty-four miles," I said. He knew exactly how much pain I was still having and that this was my first day off crutches, but I considered it a sign of progress in our doctor–patient relationship that he did not laugh out loud.

I'm surprised I didn't laugh. Training for a 444-mile bike race on a stationary bike is a laughable offense. No serious cyclist would ever do that. Triathletes and professional cyclists who are forced to train indoors during winter hook their road bikes onto a trainer. All I did was up my two-a-days of spin classes to three-a-days.

Over the next several weeks, I became extremely lonely. All my physical therapy, study sessions, and bike rides were solo missions. It was monotonous and draining, and the worst part was knowing it would be exactly the same tomorrow and the next day and the day after that. Most mornings, it was difficult to find the energy to persist, but I did, and every time I mounted that bicycle, I felt a rush of victory that I only get when I overcome my own desire to dial it back or give up completely. It's short lived, but the more you do it, the more powerful the feeling.

Ten days before the race, my lower left leg was still extremely puffy. It was holding so much fluid that it looked and felt like memory foam. When I squeezed it, my handprint took several minutes to fade. Nevertheless, I dug my old racing bike out of storage and dusted it down. It was a Griffen, and back in the late 2000s, it was top of the line. By 2021, it was a relic, and they weren't even making them anymore.

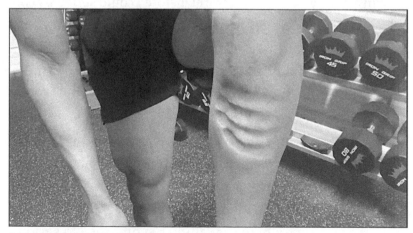

It took several months for the edema to go away.

I hooked it up to my new bike trainer and rode for two hours and eighteen minutes. In total, I completed eight sessions on the trainer. My longest ride was four hours and thirty-one minutes. But I still hadn't ridden my bike on the road when we boarded the plane for Nashville, just thirteen weeks after my surgery.

The instinct for self-preservation can make you so careful that you become reckless. My lower leg was still at least partially hollow, and I'd been through too much to expose it to distracted, impatient city drivers. I couldn't risk crashing. The Natchez Trace Parkway, on the other hand, is a smooth country road with very little traffic and no stop signs or turns, and I'd have a support vehicle. It would be as safe as road cycling gets. Unless, of course, you factored in the all-night ride and the sleep deprivation.

However, because I was hesitant to expose myself to injury, as of the morning of the race, I still hadn't ridden outside in years, I wasn't accustomed to my brand-new racing saddle, and Kish had never handed me a water bottle or food while I was on the move. So, in the few minutes we had to work with before the start of the race, Kish and I practiced the crucial exchange in an indoor parking garage.

The start was staggered, like a time trial. Every rider was on their own. I was one of the last to set off, and the early miles were a bit awkward as I relearned how and when to shift gears, but I soon settled onto the Natchez Trace Parkway, a scenic highway steeped in American history that unfurled like a smooth, undulating ribbon from Nashville, Tennessee, to Natchez, Mississippi. It rolled past creeks and swamps, traced the original trails used by merchants, explorers, and Native Americans, and skirted old indigenous ceremonial sites and trading posts. Mossy old live oaks arched and leaned over the two lanes from both directions, but I didn't notice any of that. I was busy focusing on that white line as I hammered all day without a break, and by the time I crossed the Mississippi state line, I was in fourth place.

I got through over two hundred miles in just under twelve and a half hours without much more than a pee break, but as the sun set, it became harder to ignore the withering pain in my leg. It was caused by the placement of that metal plate, which pinched the hamstring attachment. I felt it every time my leg bent, and when you're riding a bike for hundreds of miles, your leg bends an awful lot. When it finally became intolerable, I stopped in a turnout where Kish could roll up beside me.

"This was a bad idea," I muttered. "This was just dumb." I climbed into the car, dragging my leg, annoyed that I'd put myself in yet another agonizing situation. I had only officially decided to go through with the race ten days earlier and hadn't trained properly for it. I'd been doing spin classes for a few months and put in eight monotonous rides on a bike trainer while I watched ESPN. And yet, I'd still managed to ride two hundred miles. Put that way, it sounded like quite an accomplishment. More than enough to begin to convince me to pack it in. I closed my eyes and tuned in to the voice in my head. The one that is just fine with good enough.

Two hundred miles! Who does that? Who rides two hundred miles thirteen weeks after major leg surgery? You're a bad dude, Goggins!

It was all true, except that during a 444-mile race, nobody hands you a merit badge for finishing less than half of it. A better question would be, *Who rides 444 miles thirteen weeks after surgery?*

That sounds like a pipe dream, I know. That's what I thought when I opened the car door and climbed aboard my old Griffen war horse once again. I didn't think I'd last much longer, which is why my choice probably won't make any sense at all to most people. They'll consider it boneheaded to risk aggravated injury trying to finish the impossible. But Dr. Gomoll had assured me that I was not at risk of doing any damage to my knee and that the plate was secure. Plus, I know what we are all capable of when we are willing to think unreasonably and push past the point where almost everybody else would beg to stop.

The pain wasn't going anywhere. It came down to how much I was willing to endure. I thought about that when a few miles down the road, in the darkness of night, my North Star pushed aside two clouds, and Goggins rose from the ashes for the first time in almost a year.

Who rides 444 miles thirteen weeks after surgery? I do!

I rode myself into a trance. Half the time, I didn't even realize Kish was still behind me. I just followed that white line and kept cranking past all the historic roadside attractions and into the ghost world of runaway slaves and slave traders, Native American warriors, Civil War soldiers, and Lewis and Clark, and in my mind, I erased it all. I was writing a new history of the Natchez Trace. It was about the baddest person that ever came through that land on two wheels.

With about eighty-five miles to go, it started to rain. I'd been riding on carbon fiber wheels all day and stopped to switch them out for aluminum wheels. I was still in fourth place, and by then, I knew I could manage the pain and that I'd make it to Natchez. I set out again at a comfortable pace and immediately noticed how much better I felt with the new wheels. I always preferred aluminum wheels and now remembered why. They were heavier and gave me an immediate return. I could feel the power I put down with every stroke and fed off that. I had no idea how far behind the leaders I was until I flew around a bend and onto a straightaway where I saw the next two riders up ahead, a few hundred yards apart.

I breezed past them both with ease and accelerated all the way home. I was the fastest rider in the field over those final eighty-five miles and crossed the finish line on the banks of the Mississippi River in second place after riding 444 miles in twenty-five hours and change. The winner had trained for twelve months and finished just over three hours ahead of me. My first ride had been eleven weeks before race day. I was only seven weeks off of crutches and still couldn't walk without a limp.

There wasn't any time to celebrate. I'd taken a few days off from my studies to get the race in, and as soon as I'd slipped my bike into its travel case, I cracked my textbook. That massive effort on the bike was already in the rearview because I could not fall behind. I studied at the airport and on the flight home, and within eight weeks, I graduated from my Advanced EMT course as valedictorian.

In December, my attention shifted to the national exam. I stayed up until two in the morning for ten nights straight taking practice test after practice test. I answered over four thousand questions, and whenever I got something wrong, I cracked the books to understand why. I didn't like doing it, but it's not easy for me to learn, so that's the effort I must put in to be successful in the classroom.

Most people who are lagging behind in school, work, or athletics aren't willing to do what it takes to catch up and maximize their potential. They don't outwork their classmates and competitors and simply meet the standards set by their teachers and coaches. They work enough to get that passing grade and then high step it into mediocrity and convince themselves that they did their best with what they had. But I have a high bar when it comes to defining effort and success, especially in the medical field, where guesswork won't fly. Every incorrect answer on my practice tests represented someone's life ruined or lost. This wasn't a game or a sport to me. This was real world, and I wasn't looking to pass and get certified so I could go out and perform my job adequately. Which is why even after I passed my boards, I went home that night and studied those few questions that I thought I missed until I knew them all by heart.

In January 2022, I followed my North Star into the frosted upper reaches of British Columbia south of the Yukon border to explore the opportunity I'd long coveted. I met with a few senior members of the North Peace Smokejumpers in Fort St. John. It was thirty degrees below zero, the winds were howling, and the sky looked angry as they showed me around. I learned that most of the fires they deal with are caused by lightning strikes deep in the hostile wilderness miles from the nearest road, where few, if any, surveyors have ever been. Before I left, they encouraged me to apply. If I was accepted and made it through their arduous six-week training, which was set to begin in April, the workload promised to be intense.

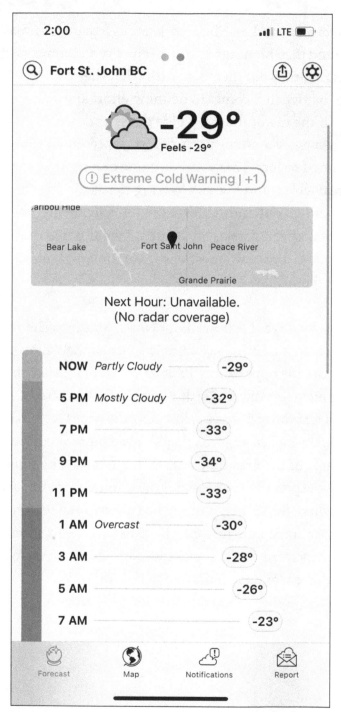

A warm welcome to Fort St. John

When my flight took off the following morning, the sky was clear enough to reveal the immensity of the landscape. There were layered mountains, granite peaks, and hundreds of miles of boreal forest rolling toward Alaska. I imagined dropping into it, and how terrifying and thrilling it would be, but the truth was I hadn't jumped out of a plane in years, I still hadn't run a lick in ten months, and Dr. Gomoll said that the one thing I supposedly could not do on my surgically repaired leg was land under a parachute.

You can work your tail off for decades, adapt, and evolve more than most, but no matter who you are or what you've done before, you cannot force something to fit. This time, even I had to admit that the odds were insurmountable. I'm often asked how I'd feel if my body rebelled and I could no longer run, ride my bike, or compete in any sport. It's an easy answer because I already know what I'd do. It might take a few months for me to work through my frustration and recalibrate, but then, I'd go be great at something else.

It had been six months since the surgery, and we were now less than two months away from my 4x4x48 Challenge, and I needed to see how it felt to run. While I'd been doing the 4x4x48 on my own for years, in 2020, I invited the people who followed me on social media to join me in the Challenge and encouraged them to push themselves a little harder while raising money for the charity of their choice. The point is to run four miles every four hours for forty-eight hours for a grand total of forty-eight miles. Over the past three years, we've collectively raised several million dollars for charities around the world. It's an honor to reflect on the impact this Challenge has had in just a few years. Countless lives have been changed or influenced by the funds raised and the experience of grinding through a single sleep-deprived weekend. That's the kind of thing that can happen when a group of well-intentioned individuals who want to be better come together to train for life.

Although it was hatched as a running event, since the beginning, I've made it clear that if running isn't possible, participants can walk, swim, or work out in the gym for about forty minutes every four hours. In 2021, in the wake of my initial knee surgeries, I couldn't run either. So I devised a high-intensity circuit workout that made running four miles feel like a spa treatment.

My goal was to run in 2022, just to see what was possible. In the second week of January, I stepped onto a treadmill for the first time in ten months for a run-walk workout. I ran for three minutes and walked for two and lasted five cycles. My left shin ached like crazy, but I continued to run every day and built up the mileage from there. Over the next several weeks, I took my running from the treadmill to the trails and finally to the streets while periodic updates from Fort St. John arrived via email.

Each one felt like a tease. Whenever I read about the physical fitness required and the tasks that awaited new recruits, I felt a flush of envy. But when I googled aspects of the training, I knew my leg was not up to the task.

In the meantime, I took a job as an emergency-room medic in a big-city hospital on the wrong side of town. We were always busy and saw patients from all walks of life. I did my best to make myself indispensable during my twelve-hour shifts, and the care we delivered was top-notch. I tapped veins for IVs, cleaned up patients with ulcers on their skin and bloody stool dripping down their legs, and helped treat others who suffered cardiac arrests. When my patient flow slowed, I scrubbed down treatment areas and cleaned the workstations. You'd never catch me sitting down unless it was my lunch break. And before and after work, and on my off days, I trained and continued with my physical therapy.

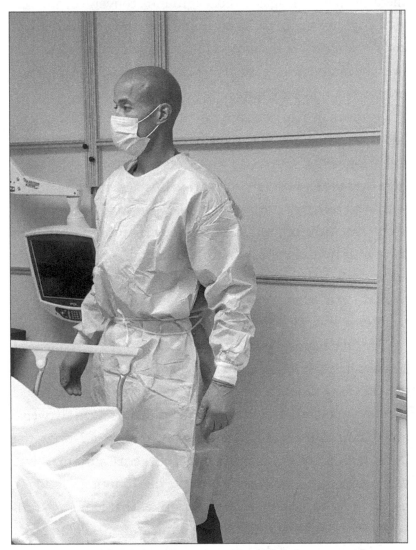

Doing rounds in the emergency room

I managed to complete the 4x4x48, and instead of leading everyone through it on Instagram Live, we took it out on the road and led several in-person group runs. The first event was in Chico, California; next was Sacramento, and we moved south from there. People of all ages and backgrounds converged, and like wild dogs, we ran in packs on singletrack trails and suburban and city streets. For the second-to-last leg, we more or less took over the famous bike path in Hermosa Beach. As the weekend progressed, I only got faster.

As much as I appreciated the turnout and enthusiasm up and down the coast, I'm an introvert, and being the center of attention is not natural for me. After a thousand selfies and high fives in Hermosa, we drove on to Costa Mesa, and I turned within to recharge during the ride. I also conducted a quick body scan. Although I still felt some burn in my left leg, I'd run forty-four miles in less than forty-one hours, was pleasantly surprised at how it was holding up, and knew I still had more to give. I was setting a new gold standard for HTO recovery. I wondered what Dr. Gomoll would say about that.

The final segment was my fastest run of all. I was challenged by several people who may or may not have run every leg. That was the thing about the weekend. Some people came out to feel the energy and ran just once in forty-eight hours. I ran all twelve, and that final one was my fastest of the weekend. During the last half mile, I wasn't even in sunny Southern California. I was way up north, where there is nothing but mountains and forests lit up by backcountry lightning strikes that have forged an airborne firefighting unit capable of meeting challenges that would make some of the hardest people I've ever met question their own toughness.

I was kidding myself, of course. Smokejumpers in Canada

don't use Ram-air parachutes, which allow for feathery land-ings. They prefer to land hard and roll. Dr. Gomoll was probably right: if I landed like they did, my leg would likely snap into at least two pieces. But every statistician will warn you that whenever you deal in probabilities, there will be outliers.

Always!

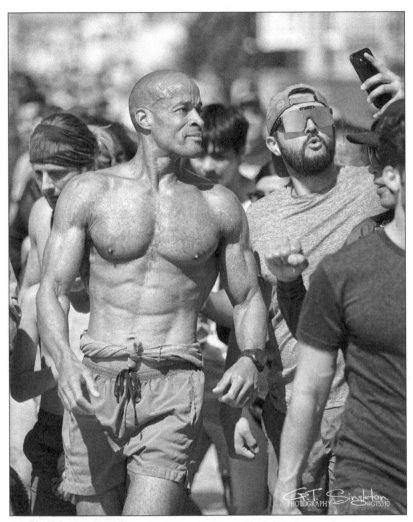

4x4x48 2022 in Hermosa Beach, an intimate run with eight hundred people.
Photo by: Jerry Singleton (@gts310)

EVOLUTION NO. 8

Most people live their whole lives without ever contemplating what it means to be great. To them, greatness looks like Steph Curry, Rafael Nadal, Toni Morrison, Georgia O'Keeffe, Wolfgang Amadeus Mozart, or Amelia Earhart. They put all the greats on a pedestal but think of themselves as mere mortals. And that's exactly why greatness eludes them. They turn it into some untouchable plane, impossible for almost anybody to reach, and it never even crosses their mind to aim for it.

No matter what I'm doing or which arena I'm engaging in, I will always aim for greatness because I know that we are all mere mortals and greatness is possible for anyone and everyone if they are willing to seek it out in their own soul. In Gogglish terms, greatness is a state of letting go of all your faults and imperfections, scavenging every last bit of strength and energy, and putting it to use to excel at whatever you set your mind to. Even if someone out there told you it was impossible. It is a feeling pursued by those rare souls willing to extend themselves beyond reason and pay the cost.

In the late 1950s, Captain Joseph Kittinger was a pilot in the Air Force tapped for experimental aviation and skydiving duty in New Mexico. He wasn't a household name. In fact, hardly anybody knew the first thing about him until August 16, 1960, when he donned a red, duct-taped pressure suit and boarded an open-sided gondola tethered to an onion-shaped helium balloon. He flew that rig nearly twenty miles high until he reached the thin atmospheric line where everything goes from blue to black. He'd traveled to a place where the horizon did not exist. He was above and beyond all previously known limitations. Suspended at 102,800 feet, he unclipped his harness and stepped into space. His free fall lasted nearly five minutes. His maximum velocity was 614 miles per hour. He plummeted over eighty thousand vertical feet before his primary chute opened. This was no Red Bull sponsored party. It wasn't a television show. Kittinger wasn't an entertainer, he was an explorer. A seeker of a new realm for the world—his flight and his jump helped make manned space flight possible—and also for himself.

I don't jump to earth from outer space, but I know that atmospheric line between blue and black. It is the glimmer of greatness that runs right through the human soul. We all have it. Most of us will never see it because to get there requires a willingness to extend yourself to the limit without any guarantee of success.

Then again, success is just another mile marker on the journey. Landing the jump and walking away while lighting a cigarette as if it were a typical day on the job made Kittinger look cool, but it didn't make him great. His willingness to do it in the first place knowing that the chances of failure were high and everything it cost him made him great. It wasn't a stunt to garner fame or publicity. It was merely an attempt to see what was humanly possible.

Just as words can be redefined, never doubt that we can redefine ourselves. It can feel impossible at times because we live in a world filled with arbitrary boundaries and fixed social lines that are as thick as the walls around a fortress. Worse, we allow those walls to limit us in too many ways. The brainwashing starts early, and it starts at home. The people we grow up with and the environments we grow up in define who we think we are and what we think life is all about. When you're young, you can only know what you see, and if all you are ever exposed to are lazy people, content with mediocrity or who convince you of your own worthlessness, greatness will remain a fantasy.

If you live in the ghetto or in a dying industrial or farming town, where buildings are boarded up, addiction runs rampant, and the schools are a mess, that will factor into the possibilities others envision for you and you envision for yourself. But even privileged people can feel shackled by their circumstances. The vast majority of parents don't know what greatness looks like, so they are ill-equipped and afraid to encourage big dreams. They want their children to have security and don't want them to experience failure. That's how limited horizons get passed down from generation to generation.

Should we really be surprised that almost everybody has a knack for twisting their story to work against themselves? I hear it all the time. Privileged kids say, "I have too much, so I cannot develop the skills that you have." The kid that came from nothing will tell me, "I don't have enough. Therefore, I cannot develop the skills that you have." No matter where someone is in life, they never fail to confess why they can't get where they need to go. The minute they open their mouths, I see how limited their horizons are, and their sob stories come with the expectation that I will deliver a "become great" package to their front door. But that's not how it works.

Identity is a trap that will keep you in blinders if you let it. Sometimes, identity is what we are saddled with by society. Other times, it's a category we claim. It can be empowering to associate yourself with a particular culture, group, job, or lifestyle, but it can also be limiting. If you stick with your own too closely, you will be susceptible to groupthink, and you may never learn who you really are or what you can accomplish. I know people who were so obsessed with landing a specific job that once they settled in to that role, they clipped their own wings. They never moved on or attempted to try anything new, and that blocked them from evolving and developing new skills.

Sometimes, we are misled by others who categorize us based on what they perceive as our identity. When I met with Navy recruiters, several tried to steer me away from SEAL training and into a different opportunity because I didn't fit the mold. I was overweight, my ASVAB scores were low, and there was my skin color. Remember, I was only the thirty-sixth Black Navy SEAL. The recruiters weren't trying to hurt me, and I don't believe they were racist. They honestly thought they were helping me by presenting more realistic options.

Usually, however, we mislead ourselves. Those of us who are struggling with our self-worth, like I was as a child, often build identities around the very things that haunt us the most. Not because we want to, but because subconsciously, we are convinced that is how everyone else sees us. You cannot allow what someone else may or may not think about you or the issues you're dealing with to stop your progress.

My environment and my history made me overanxious and stressed out. The color of my skin made me a mark. I was pre-judged and vulnerable at almost every turn, and it was my job to defy all of that. No matter how troubled or hopeless or sheltered your environment is, it is your job, your obligation, your duty, and your responsibility to yourself to find the blue-to-black line—that glimmer—buried in your soul and seek greatness. Nobody can show you that glimmer. You must do the work to discover it on your own.

There are no prerequisites to becoming great. You could be raised by a pack of wolves. You could be homeless and illiterate at thirty years old and graduate from Harvard at forty. You could be one of the most accomplished people in the country and still be hungrier and work harder than everybody else you know as you attempt to conquer a new field. And it all starts with a com-mitment to looking beyond your known world. Beyond your street, town, state, or nationality. Beyond culture and identity. Only then can true self-exploration begin.

After that comes the real work. Fighting those demons every morning and all day long is maddening. Because they only ever want to break you down. They don't encourage you or make you feel good about yourself or your long odds as you fight through all the toxic mold and crust that is self-hate, doubt, and loneliness. They want to limit you. They want you to sur-render and retreat back to what you know. They want you to quit before you get to pliability, where the sacrifice, hard work, and isolation that felt so heavy for so long become your haven. Where after struggling to visualize greatness for years, it is effortless. That's when momentum will gather like an updraft and send you airborne and spiraling toward the outer limits of your known world.

It's time to level-up and seek out that blue-to-black line. The line that separates good from great. It is within each one of us. #GreatnessIsAttainable #NeverFinished

CHAPTER NINE

WRINGING OUT THE SOUL

My eyes snapped open six minutes before my alarm started chirping. Sometimes, 0530 comes even earlier than that sounds. In my SEAL days, I woke up before the sun to take souls and wasted no time getting after it. But that April morning, I had to will myself to move an inch at a time. My left side was bruised purple from my hip to my ribs. My intercostal muscles were sore enough that even breathing hurt. My neck was so stiff that I could barely turn my head.

We were two weeks into smokejumper rookie training and deep into ground school, and it was Parachute Landing Falls (PLF) season in Fort St. John. For most of the day, my old, broken body would be bouncing off the frozen ground over and over again.

I palmed my vibrating phone from the nightstand and peeled myself off the mattress. I hadn't felt this exhausted and sore since I was twenty-four years old. Back then, I did whatever it took to lose the weight and make it through SEAL training because I knew that would change everything. I'd be able to leave Indiana behind, gain self-respect and confidence, and infuse my life with meaning. But now, there was literally nothing riding on this. I hadn't even told many people where I was or what I was doing. I had zero external motivation and all of the pain.

Every morning, I asked myself the same question. *Why am I putting myself through this?* I wasn't lacking in self-confidence or in search of meaning, and I didn't need a paycheck. Simply put, this is just who I am.

I could practically hear my bones creak as I stood up slowly, shuffled to the window, and pulled back the curtain. Another foot of snow had fallen overnight, and it was still coming down heavy. We'd expected it to be cold in Northern British Columbia, but this was something beyond. It was the coldest spring they'd had in as long as anyone could remember. When it wasn't raining, it was snowing, and the shifting north winds had a way of cutting you to the bone.

There was a time when all it would take was a hard rain pelting the roof above my bed at 0100 to ignite the savage in me. I took nasty weather like a taunting. It stripped away the gauzy fog of sleep and lit a fuse. The harder it rained or snowed, the longer I'd run because I knew that nobody would ever do something that miserable if they didn't have to. Some of my favorite runs of all time were the twenty-milers I strung out along Lake Michigan during the notorious Chicago winters, but that was some time ago.

I glanced over at Kish, all cozied up and sound asleep. Technically, I wasn't required to report to the base until 0800, and that bed was reaching out and tempting me back into her arms, so I turned to that window again and watched the snow fall. It looked to me like hell had frozen over, and that was my cue. I suited up in a thermal top, regular running shorts, and a beanie, slipped on a pair of heated gloves, and went out for a nine-mile run.

I didn't want to. The pain in my left leg was medieval first thing in the morning, but I didn't have any wiggle room. I wasn't on my own schedule anymore. For the past seven years, I'd been able to train when I wanted to. I could schedule everything else around my runs and gym workouts to optimize my fitness and performance. Now, I was a grunt again, and I could not afford to turn up at the base too stiff to function.

Those early morning runs were non-negotiable for this forty-seven-year-old rookie because almost everybody else in my rookie class was in their early or mid-twenties. Most of them came from backwoods Canada and grew up playing ice hockey six months a year. They had opted out of Generation Soft, and a handful were determined to race against me with everything they had. I respected that, but if you come for the old head's crown, there will be some push back.

Which is a long way of saying that it didn't matter if my body couldn't bounce back like theirs. Or that I had to eat cleaner food, stretch in the morning and at night, and prioritize recovery. It didn't matter if I had to sleep less because there are only so many hours in a day. If that's what it took, I was a willing warrior.

Willing warriors don't reach for excuses. While it's human nature to try and talk yourself out of doing the hard or inconvenient thing, we know that it's non-negotiable. There are a lot of people out there who are willing to sign up for the military or police force, apply for a job, or enroll in college or graduate school because they expect some tangible and timely return on their investment. Warriors aren't in it for cash or benefits. That's all gravy. Even though I was broke, I would have found a way to pay the U.S. Navy to be a SEAL. Nobody recruited me to Fort St. John, and I lost money by taking the job. But willing warriors seek out our own missions and pay any and all tolls required. I wanted to do this job, period.

It was freezing, and I was sore, but my bruises and that nasty weather didn't give a damn about me, and rest assured, that feeling was mutual. Because I was not content to just show up hoping to graduate. When you're on the older side of the age spectrum, you often get more credit than you deserve for simply showing up to do something physically challenging. Nobody expects much from you, and the temptation is there to perform to those very low expectations. Showing up is an important first step, but if you plan to show up, you may as well show out.

Nothing had been plowed yet. I bashed through powder on the feeder streets to reach the highway, where I ran in fresh, slushy tire tracks laid down by pickup trucks and big rigs. Fort St. John is populated by early risers who work on local ranches, in the oil and gas industry, or in the endless acreage of spruce and northern pine forests, and they love to drive fast on that icy highway.

My feet numbed out pretty quick, and the snow intensified to near blizzard conditions. Snow and ice pelted my face as I squinted and ran into oncoming traffic. Often, I had to dash from the middle of the road to the safety of the deeper snow on the shoulder, and whenever I was able to catch a glimpse of the driver, I found inspiration in their wide eyes of wonder and shocked expressions at having watched me materialize from the snowstorm, like a creature from another realm, a halo of steam pouring off me. They all seemed to be asking themselves the same question: "Is he crazy, or is that the most driven guy I've ever seen?"

Every footprint on that highway and each street I ran down belonged to me. Nobody else in town was out on foot. Most of the other rookies were still fast asleep. But beatdown at forty-seven years old after all I'd accomplished, I was still getting the same double takes I got back when I was in my mid- to late twenties. And that lit me up like a torch.

My injuries no longer mattered. The pain that awaited me in rookie training in just a few hours made no difference to me at all. My body was warming up, and my mind was hardening into cast iron yet again. It took close to nine miles, but the savage was ready for whatever the powers that be had planned.

The two fastest runners in class when it came to the shorter distances were a guy I called Prefontaine (PF) and another nick-named Hard Charger (HC). Both were in their early twenties, and on day one of training, when we went through a string of fitness tests, they beat me on the mile-and-a-half sprint. No one knew yet that I was just nine months out of surgery with a plate in my leg. Or that my time of 8:25 was only fifteen seconds off my personal best, set when I was a teenager in the Air Force. I was stoked with my performance. They were great athletes. To know that I was their parents' age and still able to hang with them was a reminder that I was still as hard as woodpecker lips.

A lot of the PT we did came with unknown distance and time because when fighting a fire, you never know when the exertion, the work, or the suffering might end, and the instructors wanted to see how our minds and bodies responded to the unknown element. That was tailor-made for me. The longer the run, the heavier the pack, the more intense the gym session, the greater the suck, the better I got. Those young guns may have been faster on the short course, but I almost always outlasted them.

On one ruck, HC and I broke free from the group. I pushed the pace, and he stayed on my shoulder. We were running flat out, and after a few miles of hard running, his breath turned rusty and thick. He sounded like a bulldog in heat but refused to let me drop him and was unwilling to stop. He'd stopped once before at the end of a different long run we'd done together after work. This time, he made it to the finish line, breathing like his lungs were flipping inside out, and we finished side by side, both of us spent. I turned to him, nodded, and said, "That's what I'm talking about."

I was proud of him, but I was also proud of myself. I'd had a minimal amount of time to get in shape to qualify for one of the hardest jobs in the world. It had been a demanding journey, with agony an ever-present shadow. Yet at thirteen weeks post-surgery, I rode my bike 444 miles. At eight months, I ran forty-eight miles in forty-five hours, and at nine months, I was challenging twenty-somethings in everything from running to rucking to pull-ups to hauling heavy gear a very long way. But I wasn't out to take their souls. This young group inspired me. I wanted to push them like they were pushing me because they were the next generation of hard, and though I did like winning my fair share of runs and workouts, I liked it even better when they got me.

When I arrived at work after my nine-mile run, I took one look at my classmates, and it was obvious that we were all suffering. I was the most experienced medic on the base, and some of them came to me for help with shin splints and stress-fracture symptoms. One had been concussed, and all of us had sore necks because when you are falling from three to four feet with a helmet on, your neck muscles get worked.

Morale was low. Everyone was dragging, and our esprit de corps was nowhere to be found when we were instructed to line up and start hammering out push-ups. Smokejumping requires a lot of upper body and core strength. The jumping and landing are physically demanding; plus, we would have to ruck with at least sixty pounds of hose on our backs, as well as chainsaws, pumps, and various other fire equipment—none of it light. Oftentimes, we'd be hauling water pumps and moving logs with no vehicle support. It's on us to take any gear air-dropped for us and move it into the proper position. To help prepare us for that, the instructors unleashed a steady onslaught of push-ups throughout training, among other strength-building workouts and calisthenics. There was no telling when or how many we'd have to do each day. We just knew they were coming, all day long.

That morning, our form and cadence were all over the place. Some of us hammered them out with ease. Others suffered and were clearly demoralized. After we finished, I gathered the group and told them that when it came time for the next set, we were going to do it differently and work together.

A short while later, when one of the instructors called for push-ups, everyone waited for me to hit the floor first.

"Ready!" I yelled, once I'd assumed the position.

"Ready!" they hollered and hit the deck. Then we began at my pace.

"Down!" I bellowed.

"One," they called back.

"Down!"

"Two!"

"Down!"

"Three!"

Sounding off in military cadences serves a few purposes. It helps you breathe, releases a shot of adrenaline, and builds up morale. To the uninformed, it may look and sound like unnecessary ra-ra-ra, but if you're part of an exhausted, physically and mentally taxed team, that kind of camaraderie turns something monotonous and brutal into an empowering rite of passage. You aren't even doing push-ups anymore. You are becoming one with the team, merging with a common energy force, and that helps everyone stay on course to get through each day, each module of training. We all grew to love those push-ups!

It felt good to be at the top of the class when it came to physical training, but my struggles didn't begin and end first thing in the morning. Before beginning PLFs each day, we had to suit up in our Kevlar jumpsuits in under three minutes, and given that my body was still healing post-surgery and that everything we did was outside in below-freezing temperatures, I had some complications to deal with.

I struggled to get down on my knees, and my old friend Raynaud's was back with a vengeance because I couldn't use the heated gloves during training. My fingertips lost all dexterity within minutes. I couldn't feel them or all the little zips, straps, and snaps. So it took me longer than everyone else—and much longer than the allotted three minutes—to slip into the suit, secure my reserve chute on my chest, and cinch my ditty bag between my legs. The young guys got a kick out of watching me struggle to get dressed. For the first time, I looked my age to them, and they gave me a boatload of grief. But come PT time, they always kept their mouths shut because they knew I would be bringing the pain.

As usual, the PLFs were cruel to every one of us. The unforgiving cold made the ground harder and our bodies tense and more brittle, which magnified the misery, whether we were jumping from a twelve-inch ledge, a three-foot platform, or climbing up to a different platform, swinging out on a trapeze, and letting go. It was all about building muscle memory so we could embody what the instructors called the "proper landing attitude."

When most people jump off anything high, they have a reflex to spread their arms and legs and look down as they drop. We were taught to keep our bodies in a tight formation, feet and knees together. Pinning the legs together allows you to distribute and absorb the impact. We weren't trying to stick the landing. We'd be moving much too fast for that. We practiced hitting the ground and rolling to one side. As every jump provides different elements and conditions, we had to be comfortable rolling right and left, forward and backward, and we alternated our reps.

None of this was brand new to me because I was one of the few rookies with prior jump experience. I'd jumped from a variety of altitudes and aircraft with a reasonably wide range of gear, but I hadn't jumped on a static line since my Navy SEAL days, and it did take time for me to get my technique together. Everyone had a more-challenging side, and because I was so concerned about protecting my left leg from direct impact, my hip and ribs took a beating whenever I rolled left. I absorbed the escalating pain because Dr. Gomoll's words were still tacked to the bulletin board in my brain. If the leg wanted to break, it would have to wait for a real jump. No matter how purple and swollen I became, I wasn't about to expose that tibia on a jump from a metal platform or the arc of a janky trapeze. That probably explained my general lack of fluidity. After each PLF, the instructors critiqued our form, and the word I heard the most was "clunky."

After several days of throwing myself into the dirt, we were leveled up to the shock tower, a twenty-foot platform where we sat in a mock-up of an aircraft doorway, clipped into a stiff bungee, and practiced our exits. The exercise included a ten-foot fall arrested by a sudden snapback that delivered a kiss of mild whiplash. On one of my early attempts, I stood behind a small but athletic young woman who I call PB for pit bull because she was very friendly with plenty of fight coiled deep inside her. But when she got that smack on the back from the instructor signaling that it was her time to take that leap of faith, she froze up.

PB is as God-fearing as they come. I watched my tongue around her because profanity made her uncomfortable. Boat Crew Two Goggins would have continued cursing like the sailor he was and forced her to deal with it. And when fear paralyzed her in the middle of an evolution, he may have laughed out loud. However, while my inner savage was alive and well, I was no longer that guy. Back in SEAL training, I loved when people froze up and quit. I felt it elevated me in some way, but that was ego-driven immaturity and poor leadership. These days, I consider it my business to make everyone better, no matter the job or situation. During my interview with the North Peace Smokejumpers, I was asked to describe my best quality.

"If you hire me," I said, "everyone in my class will graduate.

That's my best quality." It wasn't an empty promise. It was an oath.

"Do you want some time?" the instructor asked.

"Yeah, I do," PB said.

One of the elements that made me want to work with this smokejumping crew was their acceptance of and respect for every individual. Although there were standards to be met and exceeded and they did push us to excel, they understood that everyone has a process to work through. However, I know from experience that more time to think would not help PB in this situation.

Watching her felt like I was seeing myself in the surf zone at the beginning of my second Hell Week, looking like a stag frozen in the glow of an onrushing eighteen-wheeler. I could tell from the vacancy in her eyes that she wasn't having much fun anymore and that this jump petrified her, but some fears must be conquered immediately. The only thing that could possibly help PB in that moment was to stop thinking, look her fear dead in the eye, and jump anyway. When she backed away and suggested I take her place, I shook my head.

"Don't do that. Stay in the door and reset." We locked eyes. "If you freeze up now, it will happen again, but up there, when it's for real. So, when you get to the door, as scary as it is, sound off to get your adrenaline going. Focus on the horizon, and when that smack on the back comes, slingshot out of here."

She nodded, determined, got into position, took a deep breath, and yelled, "Am I clear?!"

"Get ready," replied the instructor, and the instant he smacked her between the shoulder blades, PB became a cannonball.

My leadership style in Fort St. John was chameleonic. To some of my classmates, I was their medic. To others, I doled out tough love in the heat of a difficult moment. I competed with the best athletes to make them even better, and I took calls at night from those who didn't think they'd make it to graduation. But I'm not sure how many understood that I too was in danger of missing the cut because of a certain skill that I literally could not grasp.

Unlike military paratroopers, who almost always jump into terrain with few, if any, natural obstacles, smokejumpers have to land in tight drop zones (DZ). In ground school, we were taught to seek out alternates when mistakes have been made or winds shifted and that primary DZ remains out of reach. There are times when you simply can't make the DZ, and with forest in every direction, it is inevitable that at one time or another, we will land in the trees, dangling alone and with nobody coming to save us. Which is precisely why we do letdown training.

We all carried 150 feet of nylon webbing in one of our leg pockets. That was our emergency letdown line. We were taught to tie it off overhead on our canopy's high riser with a series of half-hitches, then use it to rappel down safely. Theoretically. It wasn't as easy to execute as that might sound because when you're dangling by a parachute and wearing a helmet, the angles make it difficult to see the riser you're working with over your shoulder. And just because you are caught in a tree does not mean you will stay in that tree. It's best to get down to earth ASAP. Which is why this was a timed exercise. We were to get it done in under ninety seconds on both the right and left sides come test day, or we could forget about jumping at all.

I didn't come close to making the time on my initial attempts because I couldn't feel the webbing. We must have done a dozen daily reps for weeks, but the weather stayed cold, and my hands would not cooperate. I fumbled so badly it was borderline uncomfortable for the instructors and any of my classmates who were paying close enough attention. Despite my age, everyone had the highest expectations of me. I'm supposed to be able to do anything, and I was still over thirty seconds too slow with test day looming.

Once again, my struggle was on display for all to see, but I never hung my head. Everybody stumbled on something at least once nearly every day in that training, and we all have things to work on in life. That's how it should be. When you drop your head, you are sending a direct message to your brain that you don't think you have what it takes to get better. That makes it much harder to focus and succeed. When you are working toward a goal that is important to you and things don't go your way, never let anyone see it bring you down. Don't give them the satisfaction. When your head's down, you can't see where you need to go or what needs to be done. And if you need help, ask for it. Never be ashamed of it. Yes, it was freezing. Yes, I struggled mightily, but I did not sulk. I kept my head up and got to work.

I practiced every night for hours. At first, I rigged up a simulation of parachute risers with coat hangers in my closet, and before each attempt, I let my bare hands marinate in the freezer, but they never got cold enough, so I moved the operation outside, where I could sink my hands into the snow until I couldn't feel a thing. Then, I stood at the base of a tree and tied off overhead. Kish came out to time me, bundled up in three sweaters, two parkas, and multiple winter hats.

This wasn't about conditioning my hands to the brutal cold. That would never happen because of Raynaud's. But by cranking out these reps for hours, my mind and body synced up. I knew exactly where the webbing was and what to do with it, whether I could feel it or not. I chopped three seconds off my time one night. Then, another five seconds the next. My improvement wasn't immediate or substantial. But it was steady, so I kept at it.

It was not easy to maintain a positive outlook and commitment to working and training upwards of eighteen hours every day for six weeks. There is a reason smokejumping is a young person's game. I arrived in great shape, but I was using my body in a way I hadn't in years, and the torment was unrelenting. I was also mentally worn down. This was not the most challenging training I'd been in, but it was an intense struggle because I was a lot older and no longer who I used to be.

A lot of people let a realization like that limit their future. They lose their edge and scale back their ambitions and expectations to protect themselves. They retire and quit pushing themselves into uncomfortable environments and challenging situations. Much of that has to do with the age pass down. There's a pass down for everything in life. When it comes to age, we seem to share a common misperception of how we should feel or where we should be based on a number when sometimes, the problem isn't chronological. Often it isn't Father Time that is jacking you up but his brother, Father Fatigue.

They say that you can't beat Father Time, and that may be true, but you can definitely make his brother feel your resistance, and if you are willing to outlast the headwinds of fatigue minute by minute, hour by hour, day after day, you can at least meet Father Time face to face and negotiate with him. Whenever I felt too tired or sore to get out of bed, I kept my eyes on the horizon and reminded myself that smokejumper training is temporary. Some mornings, it actually felt good to be so sore because that was a sign that I was still willing to turn myself inside out to look for that blue-to-black line and do something that spoke to my soul.

True, I was not the same David Goggins. I was a much better version. I used to think you had to be the best at everything to be great and to be a strong leader. That's not the case. The valiant one is the person who faces long odds yet continues to try. When those young studs saw me running in the snow before work, it messed with them. And when word got out that this supposedly bigger-than-life forty-seven-year-old savage was putting his hands in the snow and placing them back on the let-down line for hours, hunting a physiological adaptation, it showed them what it looks like to refuse to be denied, what it means to be never finished. It reminded them that this opportunity was special and that they probably had a lot more to give too.

I made the let-down time on test day. Not by much, but I made it. I dressed in under three minutes too, and while I didn't land or roll like a gymnast or ballerina, I proved my consistency and capability to the instructors and to Tom Reinboldt, founder of the North Peace Smokejumpers, and graduated ground school.

"I can see it doesn't come naturally," Tom told me later. Like me, he'd survived a tough childhood and was drifting as a young man until he found smokejumping. At twenty-seven, after a health scare, he launched his own unit and built a culture centered on respect and excellence. None of it was easy or came naturally to him either, which is exactly why I wanted to be there. "It's good you're not a natural," said Tom. "I can see your will, and I respect that."

A few days later, in early May, we were rallied for a mock-up drill. We suited up in our armored gear, which included that

Kevlar jumpsuit as well as a helmet with a grate protecting our faces, and walked to the air strip. Our first jump was scheduled for the following morning, weather depending, and our instructors wanted us to squeeze into the Twin Otter, the smaller of the two aircraft in the unit. The point of a mock-up is to get familiar with the aircraft and where and when to clip into the static line.

This bird looked well used. The tang of jet fuel wafted down the aisle and crawled into my sinuses as we loaded up, and that stirred something in me as I sat down. My pulse quickened. My skin rippled with anticipation, but it was just a drill, and after a briefing, we disembarked into a truck. That's when the instructor asked us to do it one more time.

As I reboarded the plane, I sensed that this wasn't another drill, and then spotted the pilot make for the cockpit door. They were shotgunning us. The second we were seated, the pilot fired his propellers without giving us any time to think or back out. Two minutes later, we were airborne and climbing to 1,500 feet. When we reached altitude, the designated spotter tossed out his paper streamers to estimate wind speed. I watched them unfurl in the thermals as he pointed out the DZ.

It was a bluebird day, the wind was light at three to five knots, and we arced in long loops. One by one, we stood up, made our way to the static line, got on our knees, and clipped in.

I was one of the last to jump and was calm, if uncertain, as I stuck my pin into the line and locked it. *This is it*, I thought. *This is where the leg breaks and the dream dies.* That was the plain truth, but I took comfort in getting this far. At least I'd get one jump in. And if it was my first and last, I'd better make it sing. The spotter gave me the wind drift, pointed out the DZ, and listed the hazards. The plane banked toward my exit point, and I sounded off.

"Am I clear?!" We were traveling at ninety knots, but my pulse was surprisingly smooth as I kicked one leg out the open door.

"Get ready," he said. Despite the chill, sweat tickled the back of my neck as time slowed way down until the moment the spotter slapped my back.

"Push thousand!" I yelled and used both hands to push out the door and into the sky on a static line for the first time in fourteen years. "Two thousand, three thousand, four thousand!" There is no rip cord to pull on static line jumps—unless you need to trigger your reserve, that is—and it only took about five seconds for my canopy to open with a violent tug. "Check thousand!"

I looked up and inspected my canopy for holes or twists. My suspension lines were mildly twisted, but I recognized it, pulled my risers, kicked my legs as if riding a bicycle, and rotated out in a blink. The chute filled out, and I slowed down even more.

It steered like a barge. There was an eerie delay when I toggled left or right, but I read the wind well and maneuvered into it while I fell at a rate of about seventeen and a half feet per second. That feels pretty fast as the ground rushes toward you, but I wasn't looking down. I held steady, eyes out front, and tapped the ground with my feet and knees together. I felt a bolt of pain in my left shin as I rolled right, but it didn't last.

The leg held!

An instructor ran over, breathless yet reasonably impressed. He offered a few pointers and a hand, and as I got to my feet, I found that I could not stop smiling. It wasn't that evil Goggins smile either. This one was wide and natural, and well-earned.

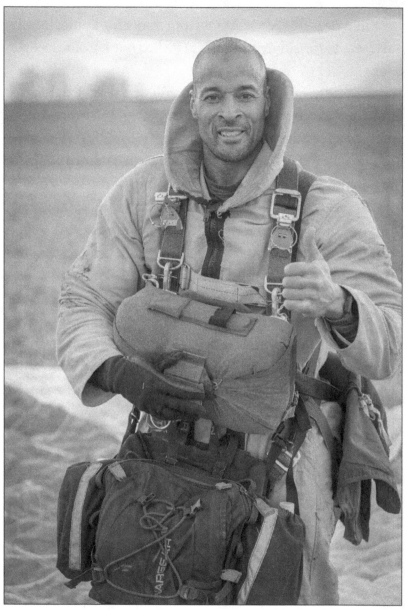

The smile is because I thought for sure the leg was going to break! (Photo by: Greg Jones)

For the next two weeks, as we kept jumping, the DZs got tighter and tighter. There were no more open fields, just tiny divots in the woods. A lot of the trees had been ravaged by beetles, but those trunks still managed to stand sentinel, like a zombie forest. From above, they looked like spikes. Those weren't the only hazards. There were boulders, rivers, lakes, bogs, downed trees, and thorny shrubs. And there were plenty of live evergreens trying to reach out and grab us too. On most jumps, at least one of our classmates got hung up. One caught the top of a ninety-foot conifer, and it barely held him. He was lucky because once his chute lost air, it was worthless, and the fall would have killed him.

There were times when the DZ was hard to make out from the bird, and the wind was wildly variable. The spotter's wind-drift intel was usually outdated within minutes, so if you weren't one of the first to jump, you'd have to figure it out on your ninety-second drop. That made it all the more difficult to avoid every hazard as I searched for the orange X laid out by the instructors.

I never got caught in a tree, but I clipped one with my shoulder on one jump, got spun around in a shifting wind, and landed hard and fast on another. It gave the instructors a scare, but I was glad it happened because once again, my leg absorbed the impact, and from then on, I knew for sure that it was good to go.

My body was healing up. The bruises had faded for the most part, and my intercostal muscles released. I could breathe free and clear by the final days of rookie training, and everything had slowed down for me. I read the wind well, steered with more confidence, zoomed closer to that X early on, and started hitting my mark with precision.

There was no pomp and circumstance come graduation, which was another sign I was exactly where I was supposed to be. A couple of the instructors said a few words, then handed us our uniforms, and that was that. All but one candidate graduated from our class, which spoke to how strong my class was and how much we came together as a team. HC looked stoked, and PB was beaming. She'd evolved from not being able to jump off a twenty-foot platform to becoming one of the very best jumpers in our rookie class.

I was proud of myself too because it had been just ten and a half months since the surgery that turned my smokejumper aspirations into mission impossible. And it had taken every ounce of endurance, dedication, and faith I had to make it. Now that I had, while it felt satisfying, I was old enough and had done enough hard-core jobs to know something that the happy young rooks did not. The hard part had just begun.

I'd seen how perilous and serious this job was. Each jump was high risk, and while we'd all been challenged to our depths, everything we had done to that point had been a mere training ground. In training, you can miss the X. You can get caught in trees. Now that we were operational, every detail had to be dialed in. On a fire, there is no time to mess around getting out of trees or hiking out of the bush in search of your crew while they wait on you. All the other rookies were smiling that afternoon. I was focused on the fight to come.

That mentality to always be looking for the next mission was a product of experience, but not only military experience. I've been discovering, developing, refining, and adapting that mindset my entire life. Many people snicker or smirk in disbelief when they watch me take on a new challenge, as if to say, "Why would anybody do that?" The implication is that I'm doing it to get noticed, to fill up on atta' boys, or for a payday. Let's make one thing clear: Before you knew me, I was a Cub Scout, a Webelo, and a Boy Scout. Before you knew me, I was in Civil Air Patrol and Junior ROTC. Then I joined the Air Force. I joined the Navy. I went to Ranger School. I went to Delta Selection. And now, I am a North Peace Smokejumper, operating from a remote airfield in Northern British Columbia. Do you think this just ends? I repeat: this is who I am!

At almost every stop along the way, there have been very few people who looked like me. I wasn't the first Black Navy SEAL, and I'm not the first Black smokejumper. Back in the 1940s, there was a team of Black smokejumpers called the Triple Nickles who fought forest fires in the American West, but their contribution was not well publicized and unfortunately is largely forgotten. Today, it is all too rare to find a Black person fighting wildfires anywhere in North America.

But it doesn't matter where you come from or what you look like, we are all hindered by supposedly fixed social lines. Whatever your gender, culture, religion, or age, there are things that you've been told your kind just does not do.

Which is why there has got to be somebody in every family, neighborhood, culture, nation, and generation who breaks the mold and changes the way others think about society and their place in it. There has got to be someone willing to be an outlier. A savage who sees those walls and barriers that are constantly trying to close us off and divide us up and then breaks them down again by showing everyone what is possible. There's got to be someone who demonstrates greatness and makes everyone around them think differently.

Why not you?

The road to success is rarely a straight line. For me, it's always been more like a maze. Many times, when I thought I'd finally cracked the code, had it all figured out, and found the straight path to certain victory, I hit a wall or got spun into a turnaround. When that happens, we have two choices. We can stay stuck or regroup, back up, and try again.

That's where evolution begins. Hitting those walls time and again will harden and streamline you. Having to back up and formulate a new plan without any assurances it will ever pan out will tune your SA up and develop your problem-solving skills and your endurance. It will force you to adapt. When that happens hundreds of times over the course of many years, it is physically exhausting and mentally draining, and it becomes damn near impossible to believe in yourself or your future. A lot of people abandon belief at that point. They swirl in the eddies of comfort or regret, perhaps claim their victimhood, and stop looking for their way out of the maze. Others keep believing and find a way out but hope to never slip into a trap like that ever again, and those skills they'd honed and developed whither. They lose their edge.

I am always on the hunt for another twisted pretzel of a maze to get lost in because that's where I find myself. The smooth road to success is of no use to savages like me. That may sound ideal, but it won't test us. It doesn't demand belief, so it will never make us great. We all build belief in different ways. I clock countless hours in the gym, where I log thousands of reps and run and ride my bike obscene distances, to cultivate belief. Despite what you may think, I don't consider myself an ultra-athlete because those races are not who I am. They are tools. Each one provides me a stockpile of faith so when I get stuck in the maze of life like a broke-down savage, I still believe I am capable of achieving my unreasonable goals, such as becoming a smokejumper at forty-seven years old, no matter what society or the good doctor says.

I don't mean to suggest that you must run one hundred or two hundred miles to believe you have what it takes to get where you want to go. That's what I had to do based on the depth of the darkness I came from and the scale of my ambitions. But if you've lost it, you do need to find your way back to belief. Whatever it takes for you to believe that you're better than good enough to achieve your dreams is what you must do. And remember, your greatness is not tied to any outcome. It is found in the valiance of the attempt.

My crew was one of four on standby when the winds picked up and thunderheads blew across Northern British Columbia. We were on our satellite base in Mackenzie when the call came in mid-morning that there had been a lightning strike and a three-acre fire was burning outside of Fort Nelson. Although I'd graduated rookie training, you aren't officially a smokejumper until you jump your first fire, and I was about to be baptized. Our three-man crew hopped into the DC-3—a refurbished World War II relic—with three other crews, enough firefighting gear to put the burn down, and two days of food and water.

We flew for ninety minutes until we reached the billowing black smoke, and leveled off at 1,500 feet. The streamers flew, and the spotter pointed out an overgrown pipeline corridor, no more than twenty feet across, roughly a quarter mile from the flames. That was the DZ. Kneeling in the open doorway, the spotter shouted the wind drift and the hazard rundown over the roar of the propellers. *Roger that*, I thought.

"Am I clear?!" I hollered.

The plane rattled and shook. It was so loud, I could barely hear myself think. My pounding heart sent a flood of adrenaline rocketing through me. Locked into the static line, I stepped to the door, grabbed the outside edges with both hands, and flung myself into the sky in time to watch a teammate's parachute bloom 150 feet below me. Once my chute opened, the rumble of the propellors and wild hiss of the wind melted to a peaceful whisper. I looked down, located my DZ, identified all the hazards, and took in the full scope of the fire. There was danger in every direction, yet all I saw was beauty.

My body had failed me for eight years straight. I could have given up a dozen different times at least. Many late nights and early mornings, my doubt was louder than that DC-3. I had to sit with that doubt, stare into it, and, more often than not, I had no answers, no good reason to think I would ever get here because I kept falling short for one reason or another. It's easier to overcome doubt that you've built up in your mind. It's much harder when you know you've failed more than once and that the odds of success are slim. But because of the way I live and thanks to the mindset I work hard to cultivate, I had enough belief left to try one more time.

Nothing in my life has ever happened for me on the first try. It took me three cracks to get through Navy SEAL training. I had to take the ASVAB five times and failed twice before breaking the Guinness World Record for most pull ups in twenty-four hours. But by then, failure had long since been neutralized. When I set an unreasonable goal and fall short, I don't even look at it as failure anymore. It is simply my first, second, third, or tenth attempt. That is what belief does for you. It takes failure out of the equation completely because you go in knowing the process will be long and arduous, and that is what we do.

I wish I could more fully express what it's like to defy the medical mind to parachute into wildfires at forty-seven years old. I find the sensation almost impossible to describe. All I can say is that I hope you and everyone else get to feel this one day because to overcome all obstacles and bump up against the outer reaches of your capabilities is the pinnacle. In those rare, fleeting moments when you are washed in the sense of infinite possibility and overwhelmed with glory, everything they ever did to you or put in front of you—all of the disrespect, knockdowns, and breakdowns, and every bit of the pain, doubt, and humiliation—is worth it. But the only way to get there is to continually seek greatness and always be willing to try one more time.

I never needed to be the hardest person in the world. That became a goal because I knew it would bring out my best self. Which is what this messed-up world needs from all of us: to evolve into the very best versions of ourselves. That's a moving target, and it isn't a one-time task. It is a lifelong quest for more knowledge, more courage, more humility, and more belief. Because when you summon the strength and discipline to live like that, the only thing limiting your horizons is you.

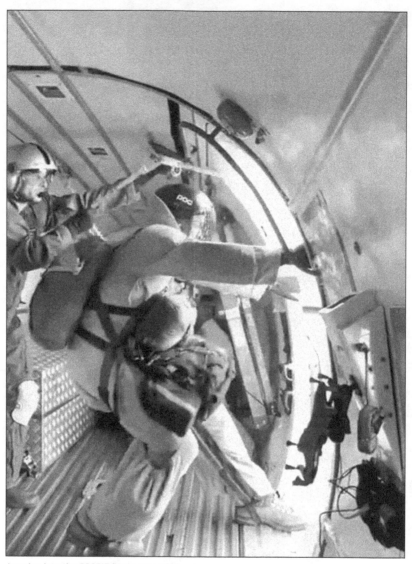

Jumping into the G90317 fire in June 2022

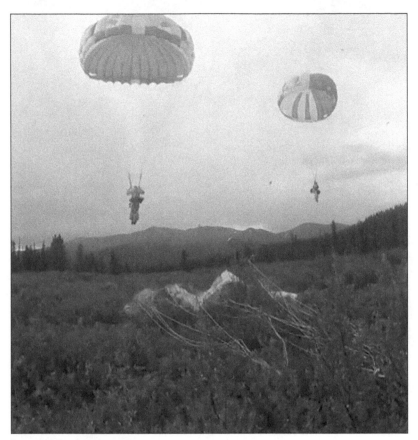

Second fire jump of the season

ACKNOWLEDGMENTS

To Jennifer Kish, who would do whatever it takes to help me reach my outer limits. You have been around for some of the most difficult times that I ever had to endure. Thank you for showing your steady hand. You have redefined what "ride or die" means.

Adam Skolnick: Thank you for showing up every day with an open mind and the attitude required for setting a new bar that will be impossible for many to achieve. This book is one for the ages.

Jacqueline Gardner: Like always, Mom, my thank-yous can only truly be understood by you. If only he could see us now! Neither one of us turned out the way he said.

Dr. Andreas Gomoll: Many more chapters of my life will be written because of your work. It will end one day, but not today.

JeVon McCormick and Scribe Media: JeVon, in a world of crooked people always looking for an angle, I thank you and your team for having character. The character to take care, not take advantage, of each and every one of your clients. The work you all do is second to none.

Joe Rogan: Your friendship and support have been very meaningful throughout the years. It shows what kind of a man you are that you not only believe that there is enough success for everyone but do your part to help facilitate that for others. It takes a rare combination of confidence and security to be willing to do that.

Dwayne "The Rock" Johnson: When it comes to big-time celebrities, you are the example that others need to follow. Your humility speaks volumes about your character. Saying "Stay hard" to you is wasted breath. Stay real, DJ!

Tom Reinboldt: You created a special culture in a world where humility is all too often lost. You have built an environment that not only teaches leaders how to lead but also how to follow.

CPSIA information can be obtained
at www.ICGtesting.com
Printed in the USA
BVHW081715011222
653239BV00003B/14

9 781544 536828